MY FAMILY RECORD BOOK

The Easy Way to Organize Personal Information, Financial Plans, and Final Wishes for Seniors, Caregivers, Estate Executors, etc.

HARRIS N. ROSEN

PUBLISHER'S INFORMATION

HARRIS N. ROSEN BOOKS

EMAIL: SURVIVORINFO@AOL.COM
WEB: WWW.SURVIVORINFORMATION.COM

ISBN: 978-0-692481-6-22

Cover Design by Let's Write Books, Inc.

Paperback Book Design by
Elizabeth Rosen (elizabethrosen.com)
Design and Printing Support: (eBookBakery.com)

Writing Coach - Lisa Tener (lisatener.com)
Editing - Tracy Hart (editingwithhart.com)

To Myrna,
who taught me the
meaning and value of family
and helped me to be
everything I could be.

BONUS: Download the FREE
companion app at
www.MyFamilyRecordBook.com

CONTENTS

5

Part B
So Your Loved Ones Can Go
On Living!

ACKNOWLEDGEMENTS

While scores of people contributed to this book and urged me to write it, several deserve special thanks, and I am deeply grateful for all their help.

Jeff Brier, George deLodzia, Nancy Harris, Paula Izeman, and Natalie Pelavin read the manuscript and made suggestions and corrections in content, structure, and grammar. Wendy Lapides, a daughter (by marriage), did research, obtained others' opinions, reviewed websites, read the manuscript, and recommended changes resulting in accurate content.

Others provided expertise and guided me in their fields: Meyer Goldstein – attorney and expert on deferred giving, trusts, and endowments devoted his time to make me realize (not once, but *twice*) that the entire book should be reorganized. (Me? Disorganized?) And although I didn't agree at first, he kept at it, and because of his incisive analysis, the book is far better. (All the while, he was studying to reenter the bar in both Rhode Island and Massachusetts, which he accomplished.)

Ian Barnacle, who manages over 50 real estate agents, was not afraid to give constructive criticism to his grandfather; Peter Colella, my insurance advisor for a long time, reviewed that section and added tips, which I included; Jerry Dorfman, CPA, FS, my financial and tax advisor for years, provided insight, having helped many a new widow and widower understand his or her new financial role and responsibilities; Ed Feldstein, an attorney and friend, took a special interest in this book and supplied helpful information; and another daughter (by marriage), Sally Lapides, the impresario of Rhode Island real estate, read parts in Section 2 in which she is a nationally-recognized expert.

Betsy Elias, a niece, whose knowledge and experience was gained as an executive with a major U.S. publisher, encouraged my being accurate and thorough.

My daughter, Elizabeth Rosen, nationally recognized illustrator, offered guidance and designed the original outstanding covers. In spite of what your high school art teacher said, you climbed the mountain and have succeeded so well with talent he didn't recognize. I am indeed very proud of you.

Thanks to Lisa Tener and Tracy Hart, book coach and my editor, respectively. Lisa provided much of the initial encouragement and support, and Tracy had a relentless eagle eye, strengthening the book with determined suggestions, yet always reminding me that it was my book – a terrific duo from South County, Rhode Island.

Nancy Harris, Wendy Lapides, Michael McCann, Gene Mihaly, Cindy Peckham, Richard Shein, and Ronnee Wasserman tested computer directions provided as appendices and made me improve them. A friend of 75+ years, Herb Triedman, provided inspiration (and for me, perspiration) to simplify what I had written.

I am also indebted to the many friends who unfortunately became widows in the past five years and shared their personal experiences. Although some of their stories are related, their privacy is respected. They all strongly encouraged me to write this book – especially one friend who said, "Where was this book when I needed it?"

But most importantly: I am grateful to my wife, Myrna, who gave me the love, encouragement, and space to write this book, as well as a wonderful and meaningful life these past three decades.

So to all: my heartfelt appreciation. This is the book we have all created.

FOREWORD

Don't wait to plan until someone dies; then it's too late.

Consider the plight of a friend whom I shall call "Jane," who has four stepdaughters. Each has a boyfriend, all with eyes on the valuable collections of photographic goods, stamps, and model trains, belonging to Bill, her husband, who does not trust these secondhand stakeholders. If Bill dies first, how will she divide his loved possessions among dispassionate parties who will only sell them for play money? It is obvious that neither Stephanie nor Bill understand the decisions that will need to be made when one dies, nor do they appreciate the confusion, mental paralysis and depression that may accompany their loss.

This is where preplanning, organization and Harris "Hershey" Rosen come together.

My first meeting with him was as consultant to his company. Hershey wanted his supervisors to know more about planning, conflict resolution, and the role of a manager, and I was asked to do the training. In the process, I got to know his organized mind, his desire to have things in order and his caring for others. When he retired from leading a candy manufacturing firm with five plants in the New England area, I was delighted that he agreed to team-teach management courses with me at the University of Rhode Island, as his wealth of experience would add reality to the theory of the text book. It also added liveliness to the classroom as he frequently disagreed with me, and our classes became increasingly popular. In addition, he was a special assistant to the dean of the College of Business at the University, where he led a strategic planning process for the college.

Unlike books that only suggest recording digits and sometimes documenting locations into premade charts, *My Family Record Book* prompts record-keepers to state in-formation in their own words so that loved ones can continue living a productive life, and that provides an executor with unambiguous instructions. Hershey's realistic, executive management approach, drawn on years of practical experience, prepares the survivor to focus on the pragmatic necessity for order – an approach that is usable because of its sensitivity to his or her well-being.

Starting with desired funeral arrangements and ending with a helpful guide to downsizing and "getting rid of stuff," *My Family Record Book* has a panoramic view of the transition into widower- or widowhood. Hershey has simpli-fied and helped the process along, based on his sense of organiza-tion, and ability to counsel employees, clients, and students.

His thorough and personal approach has given new life to a book that had to be written, especially for people like Jane, Bill, and me.

George deLodzia
Professor Emeritus
College of Business Administration
University of Rhode Island
Kingston, Rhode Island

INTRODUCTION

If you're going through hell, keep going.
Winston Churchill

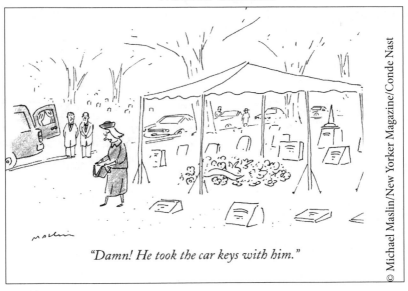

"*Damn! He took the car keys with him.*"

The Goals of This Book

The purpose of this book is to motivate your family's record-keeper, financial manager, and maintainer of the property to commit to paper the information in his or her[1] head, pertaining to the smooth functioning of your household. Possibly it is a joint effort with the record-keeper and his or her partner or loved ones to create this *Guide So Your Loved Ones Can Go On Living!* (hereafter called your *Guide*). Moreover, the book is certain to inspire deep conversations relative to end-of-life wishes.

Your *Guide* will ensure that an estate attorney spends fewer billable hours searching through a house, basement, or attic for records, contracts, warranties, and bills.

---

1. I realize that each relationship is different, and thus the references "he" or "she" or partner in this entire book are totally interchangeable.

Further, your *Guide* will result in a "Bible" your executor can use to carry out your final wishes, as your partner or executor transitions to being the person responsible for household and financial matters.

Perhaps most important, although your loved ones will need the advice of professionals (which I am not), your *Guide* will help your survivor know where he or she stands financially. They will feel that you, the record-keeper, are still there, still trying to provide protection, still trying to make life easier – at least as easy as it can be as they deal with the sorrowful task of living without you.

Comfort when it is needed the most.

So Why Is This Book Different (...from all other books)?
My Family Record Book goes beyond books, pamphlets, and CDs on the market that offer fill-in-the-blank forms. **Your *Guide* will elicit explanations that don't fit in a "box."**

For example, relative to finances, this book helps loved ones or the executor *understand* information. It prompts the record-keeper to explain in his or her own words, where assets come from, the purpose of various accounts, and how to access funds – in addition to account numbers and document location.

And merely stating the digits of our car lease and where the leases are, will not inform my wife that when one of us dies, lease payments still have to be paid until the end of the lease.

Or that there are separate monthly payments for Plan D drug coverage for each of us, but only one joint monthly payment for medical, as well as dental insurance.

And, and, and ...

However, some information is easier to comprehend when listed in a chart. Another goal of *My Family Record Book* is to assist you in generating your own tables of information.

But since the record-keeper may not be a computer whiz with Word®, **this book teaches you how to create your own blank chart or table.** 14

(See Chapter 28 and appropriate appendix.)

My Family Record Book is intended to be read and understood by you, the record-keeper; a future survivor; and your executor/executrix. Of special note are the benefits that will be gained from reading the **chapters on downsizing, getting rid of stuff, and organizing an easy relocation** (Chapters 21-24.)

Uniquely, **this book also teaches you how to establish a simple locator system.** It's not complicated and comes from my forty years of manufacturing experience in a company with five locations, covering almost 600,000 square feet of factory space – so it was necessary to know *exactly* where a given item was. (The average home is almost 2,400 square feet by comparison.)

Still, it may not be enough to say that the checkbook is in the desk. *Where* in the desk? Your description of a "location" may not be sufficient for your partner – let alone your executor – but it will **reduce stress, and save time and money,** if you learn how to identify locations of important documents (Chapters 25-27.)

Additionally, humor, true vignettes, and detailed instructions set *Creating a Guide So Your Loved Ones Can Go On Living!* apart from books of a similar nature. Won't you, the record-keeper, feel better knowing you have done everything in your power to help your loved ones into the next phase of life? I know I do.

Good luck with writing your own *Guide So Your Loved Ones Can Go On Living!*

Spouses, Partners, et al

In this book, reference is made to spouses, but I well realize that people have partners, companions, significant others, Para-kin or POSSLQs[2] - all of whom are just as important as a spouse. This book is meant for everyone, regardless of his or her relationship or legal status to the record-keeper.

---

2. POSSLQs: Persons of the Opposite Sex Sharing Living Quarters – a term established in the late 1970s by the Census Bureau. Para-kin: A term gaining popular use for individuals who co-habit, live together as a family or act as a parent, but who are not related legally.

Yes, there may be too much information in your *Guide* – more than you ever wanted to know. It is, after all, the breadth of knowledge about the mechanics and logistics of your life that your best friend had in his or her head which helped make your life what it was.

During my first week of college at Harvard, the president of the university addressed our freshman class and explained that it was not the university's purpose in the next four years to have us memorize information, but rather to learn where to get it.

The same holds true with your *Guide*. Glance through it, and familiarize yourself with the chapter headings, and then when you need to know or find something, you'll know where to look.

A word of caution: This book does not deal with family politics or even greedy hands, if they exist, but rather with the issues of running your finances and your home, as well as some pointers on downsizing. It is important for you to know whom to trust.

You can, however, feel confident that your *Guide* has been prepared with love - as a gesture to help ease you into the next phase of your life, and I hope that it does. It won't be easy; but maybe, just maybe, your *Guide* will help to facilitate that transition.

HNR

SECTION 1

Why Write a Guide?

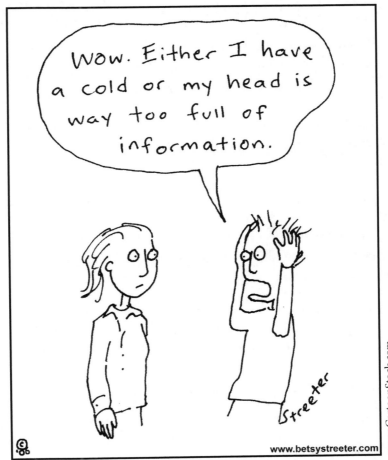

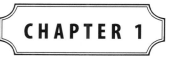

CHAPTER 1

Why I Wrote a Guide

When I retired some years ago, I had newly-found time. When people asked, "So how do you keep busy these days?" I told them of my project: writing an informational guide for my wife. "Why don't you write a book, which I could have used when Jim died? I wouldn't have felt so lost and scared."

Me? Write a book? And get it published? Sounded like a pipe dream. But here it is, and I'm pleased that you'll benefit.

The Background

For the past few decades, my wife, Myrna, and I have done our best to protect each other and provide a good life for ourselves, our family and our community. As it turns out, she is the social director, cook extraordinaire, arbiter of good taste, and of course, my best friend.

My roles? The keeper of the records, the one who handles our finances and the one who maintains our house, including its appliances. And a happy and rewarding relationship it is. But I started thinking some years ago: Who will handle all these things if I die first? How will my wife find out all the information I have in my head? Does she know:

- *Who* carries health insurance for the family and whom to contact if there's a problem?

- *What* ongoing service contracts for the house we have and where they are?

- *Where* unpaid and paid bills are?

- *When* to pay multiple year commitments to charitable organizations?

- *How* to transfer cash into her checkbook?

- And who knows what else?

Even if Myrna knew these answers (and the other million-and-one bits of information used to manage finances and our home), would she have the presence of mind (or time) to relate all this information to our executrix so she could become knowledgeable?

Myrna says I've promised her that she can go first, but you know the old adage: Man Plans and God Laughs. Still, she couldn't be less interested in all this detail. Never was and never will be – until the day it is needed.

Our executor (in our case, our executrix) will have a fiduciary as well as family responsibility, and since she won't want to make mistakes, she will engage a professional, who, naturally, will charge an hourly fee. Our executrix will know even less than Myrna, but by providing all these details, the time (and funds!) needed by the professionals should be greatly reduced.

So how could I relate to both my wife and/or our executrix not only the current information but also that which changes from year to year, such as health insurance premiums, maintenance contracts for the house and canceled or new credit cards?

Who can remember it all – especially at my age? Not me. My solution?

I started to commit this myriad of facts to paper and was amazed at how much information I needed to relate. I entered it in a Word® document on the computer and printed it out. For my wife and executrix it is in a notebook entitled, "Information for Myrna," and each page has the date on it (see Chapter 28 and the appropriate appendix), so others know when I updated it. Now, finished for the moment, I have given a copy to Myrna (who of course hasn't looked at it), and I have given copies to our executrix, estate attorney and accountant – as there's something for everyone. And our rabbi has a copy of our Chapters 4 and 5 so he knows the details of each of our funerals.

I review Myrna's guide annually or as information changes. This is not just my personality or penchant for perfection. Altered information needs to be conveyed to my partner and executrix.

A few years ago, when I was updating my "Information for Myrna," other friends, whose spouses had recently died, strongly suggested that when they became the record-keeper, life would have been much easier if they had the information that my loved ones will have. Perhaps yours should have it as well.

CHAPTER 2

Why You Should Write *Your Guide*

Yes, relating all the pertinent information you have in your head is a daunting task. Far too much to do in even a month. But that doesn't mean you shouldn't do it. So, glance through Section 2 to determine what information has to be passed on, review Section 3 to learn how to write your own Guide, and then do one or two chapters at a time. But at least get started. This chapter will tell you why.

The following stories are true.

A close friend, Anne, whose husband died a few years ago, spoke of her experience.

Although she expected his impending death, she was totally unprepared for her own reaction. Strong emotions came to the surface, she related, and things she did before without thinking became a major issue. Although a capable and accomplished businesswoman in her own right, she was almost paralyzed when it came to the seemingly-simple task of opening a checking account. Zapped of all energy, everyday tasks became formidable. Food shopping and going to the cleaners became major events. In fact, anything out of the house was a challenge.

Another friend, Lisa, didn't have any warning. The night before, she and her husband had gone out to dinner. The following morning George got up early for an appointment and went into the bathroom to brush his teeth. But he never came out.

She heard a loud thud as he slumped to the floor. In total shock and dismay, she knew instantly that she was facing the hell of her life without her best friend and trusted partner. Both hard-working, they hadn't been able to save much but were getting by and had a great marriage. Now fear and panic about her future felt overwhelming. She was petrified. Without George's income, would she have to move? How would she make ends meet? What taxes were due and when?

In another instance, a friend was helping me with the book. Ten minutes after he finished reading it, his phone rang. It was his mother – quite distraught, because her husband was in the hospital, and she knew there were bills to pay. She didn't know if there was enough money in the checking account to cover them nor did she have the foggiest idea how to transfer funds from their savings to their checking account.

Then there's what Ronald Reagan called "The Long Goodbye" – dementia, which places a spouse in the uncomfortable position of having all the financial and medical responsibilities without being able to start life again. The care-giver assumes a tremendous burden.

These are not times for the game of hide and seek - where the care-giver or survivors have to find information that seems to be hidden.

We all think we will be prepared, but close friends and my own experience tell me that death or disability of a loved one is all-consuming and totally disorienting. There may be emotional reactions of confusion, unrelenting tears, anger or panic; or physical effects, such as stomach problems, headaches or fatigue. And there might be psychological symptoms, such as needing to be in control, lost ability to trust, and feelings of isolation. Tragically, Anne and Lisa experienced it all.

Creating a *Guide* for your loved ones will empower him or her through knowledge. Your partner or executor will not be overwhelmed by the gigantic task of figuring out the logistics of home maintenance and finances.

Unfortunately, the death of a loved one may very well make a partner vulnerable to scams and fraud, even by family members – children who want an "advance" on their inheritance. Your partner or loved ones will feel secure knowing who you feel are trusted professionals pertaining to economic stability.

Likewise, a new widow or widower may receive calls from potential suitors. But as one recent widow said to me, "I don't want to be either a nurse or a purse." Your *Guide* provides freedom from needless worry and doubt about future security. (Provided, that is, that you've put your financial affairs in good order.)

Perhaps most poignantly, your *Guide* will be a conduit for your protective and loving presence. A rabbi friend tells me that people will stop calling in six to nine months, and that's when problems may occur. Indeed, the National Mental Health Association reported some years ago that: "One-third of widows/widowers meet the criteria for depression in the first month after the death of their spouse, and half of these individuals remain clinically depressed after one year." And the Harvard Medical School Family Health Guide says that: "In the year after a spouse's death, 50% of widows develop depression."

And that's why you want to make life easier for your partner and loved ones - by relating the information you know they will need to maintain the life style you want him or her or them to have.

So read on.

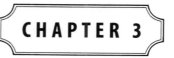

CHAPTER 3

Tips For Writing *Your* Guide

The most difficult part of writing this book was starting it.

It's amazing that when you sit down at the computer, the ideas seem to flow. Yes, I have reorganized it several times, and possibly you will redo yours, too. But once I began, it was less difficult than I thought. I hope the tips in this chapter will make it easier for you.

The purpose of this book is to make people aware of the aftermath from the loss of a loved one, and to facilitate writing your own *Guide* for your loved ones. Here's how to do it:

- First, read or skim this book to get a general idea of the information you need to impart. Then begin to write your own *Guide* by following the prompts and questions in this book. Simply type the subject heading and write your own wise words relative to your situation.

- You may find it easiest to type on a computer (be sure to print out a copy), write it down in a notebook, or even speak part of it into a tape recorder. Whichever method you use, make your loved ones aware of it.

- Keep It Simple. There's so much to tell, but try to extract the important stuff.

- Yet, do include why you have taken the actions you have, why you have engaged the professionals you have, and why all those accounts exist.

- Update it yearly. Make notes of changes throughout the year, and keep these changes on the inside cover of the notebook as a reminder for an annual update.

- As you are writing your *Guide*, think about who will receive a copy: Children? Executor? Clergy? Attorney? Accountant? Wealth advisor? Brokerage representative? Do these people know who is handling which responsibility and how to contact them?

- On which computer will your *Guide* be so that your partner or executor can update it for themselves? Is it backed-up anywhere?

- And lastly, have your loved ones and executor read the *Guide* to be sure they understand what you've written.

Starting in Section 2, it will be suggested that your *Guide* show all kinds of information in a chart or table form. Not in a premade chart as those, by definition, limit what information can be passed on. But maybe you don't know how to use Word® to create a blank chart (called a "table" in Word®)?

Neither did I.

So skip ahead to Chapter 28 and the appropriate appendix, which instruct the technologically-disadvantaged on how to do it. If that doesn't work, engage a grandchild or a local student to get you up to speed.

Chapter 28 and Appendices 1-6 have been tested by others who did not feel comfortable or competent with computers, and they were successful. Try it! You might even think it's fun.

Now on to Section 2 - the information to be included in your *Guide*.

SECTION 2

Information to Include In *Your Guide*

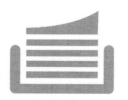

Section 2
Part A
Information Required When You Die

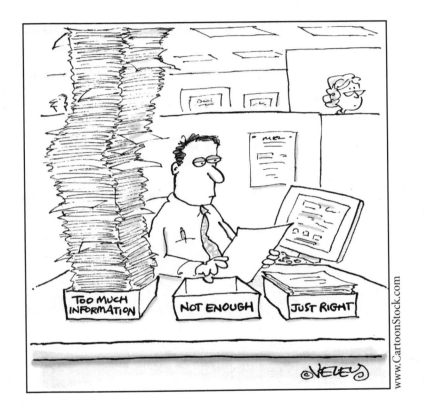

CHAPTER 4

Needed at the Time of Passing

I was very close to my mother-in-law (yes, mother-in-law). In her senior years she had been healthy, but finally started to fail at 97. It didn't matter: When the end arrived, her death knocked me for a loop. I can only imagine what the death of a spouse or partner must be like. We'll need all the help we can get, and that's where we start: what our survivors need to do first.

Anatomical Gifts

The very first question your loved ones will be asked upon your death: Is the deceased an organ donor? The next question may be: should, and may, an autopsy be performed?

How do you feel about these issues? Do you have religious objections or moral convictions? My own *Guide* says:

We have both spent our lives trying to help others, and if an organ donation will help someone else, do it and use your best judgment.

Obviously, like so many other questions to be asked, there is no right and wrong – but a decision has to be made. It may be easier to answer it now *with* your surviving spouse than his or her having to answer it later *without* you.

Calls to Be Made Immediately

The first calls made by your survivors will be to your children and/ or one or two of your closest friends to let them know what has happened. They will, most likely, provide the most comfort at a time when maximum support is needed. Oftentimes children or these friends communicate the sad news to other family members and friends. A list of family and friends could come in mighty handy, especially if this is not your first marriage. While siblings know how to contact each other, it need not be a time to figure out who else should be called and by whom.

It will also be necessary for your clergy to be notified – assuming you are affiliated with a house of worship. So another of the first entries in your *Guide* will be the name(s) of your clergy and his or her phone numbers – office, home and cell. And it would be wise to give him or her copies of this chapter and the next one of your *Guide*. Our rabbi has these two chapters for us.

If you are not so affiliated, give thought now as to what you want to happen: a funeral or memorial service, now or later? Do you know the funeral director that will handle the arrangements? If so, state the name, address and telephone numbers. If you do have clergy, perhaps he or she will handle the terrible task of contacting the funeral home.

And someone should call your attorney to be sure your loved ones don't take or omit some action that will be regretted later. (For example, forgetting to retain receipts and record all expenses related to the funeral.) So having his or her name and phone numbers for notification in this chapter, as well as in Chapter 6, is important.

Don't know this information? Collect it now since this is the first act of kindness to make it easier for your loved ones.

Calls to Others
You should also compile a list of people, and their phone numbers, to be called by combing through your personal telephone book(s), computer and PDA contacts, old party lists and personal calendars: all good sources of people to be informed. Note that my own list:

- Includes numbers for cell, office, vacation, and summer and winter seasonal phones

- Asks people to call others

- Lists calls by priority

- Suggests who makes the calls

I divided my list into two parts: immediately (yes, NOW) and later – in a couple of hours.

You may want to wait until funeral arrangements are known before making out-of-town calls, so close friends can arrange travel plans. Local people may find out through word of mouth, an organizational email, or the local newspaper obituary, so they can be called sooner.

My own list looks something as follows:

<u>People to Call</u>

Called by Mary

First Name	Last Name	Phone Number	Others This Person Should Call
Phyllis	Sinclair	xxx-yyyy	
Jen and Frank	Brown	aaa-xxx-yyyy Her cell xxx-yyyy	
Michelle	Green	xxx-yyyy	Deb Hanson
Bob	Johnson	Pvd: xxx-yyyy FL: aaa-xxx-yyyy	

Called by Barbara

First Name	Last Name	Phone Number	Others This Person Should Call
Emily and Bill	Davis	xxx-yyyy	Other cousins
Sophie and Alex	Jackson	aaa-xxx-yyyy His office xxx-yyyy	His older brother

Appointing a House Manager

Your partner will either need to be tended to or will be devoting his or her attention to kindred mourners – not to the logistics of managing the house. People, food and flowers will arrive, and someone needs to be in charge. So, your partner or survivor should appoint a "house manager" - one who can coordinate meals for the family, and record gifts and phone calls so that friends can be thanked later, and dishes and plates can be returned. Not a task for someone under a great deal of stress. So plan now. Who will it be?

CHAPTER 5

Funeral Arrangements

I have had upsetting moments in my life, but nothing prepared me for a visit to the funeral home to make arrangements for my mother. It was the first time I was in that situation, and I felt unnerved, on edge and vulnerable.

Yet decisions had to be made. I was with my father, but he was so distressed he was unable to think clearly. I vowed, right then and there, that in the future, it was important not to do this alone. And I didn't; when the time came, my sister accompanied me to the funeral home, and I felt a sense of comfort because we did it together. That's what you are doing in this chapter – making decisions as a family.

For Whom Does the Bell Toll?

The paragraphs below ask many questions, and they have to be answered not only by and for you, the record-keeper, but also for your partner (if he or she exists), so your executor knows the specifics to carry out. This is especially true if you and your partner hold different religious beliefs, with different practices and customs.

Prepaid Funeral Arrangements

If there are any such preparations, outline what these are and with whom they have been made. What is covered? What is not? What was the cost and when was it paid? Is there anything in writing? And where is that paperwork located? (See Chapters 25 - 27, which discuss how to locate documents.)

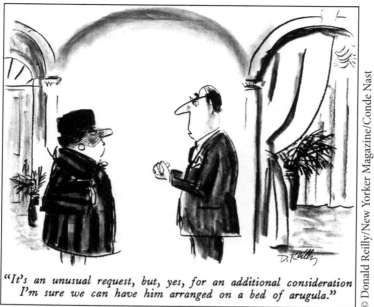

"It's an unusual request, but, yes, for an additional consideration I'm sure we can have him arranged on a bed of arugula."

Meeting with Clergy

If associated with a member of the clergy, it is with him or her that your loved ones will discuss: the time and place of the service, the funeral director to be used, the place of burial and the calling hours (Shiva or a wake). A conversation with your clergy will ensure that religious traditions are observed. And remember, there is a great deal of flexibility in what is "right" and "wrong," so discuss with clergy and other close family members your specific wishes, too.

At the Funeral Home

If there is not a prepaid contract, your loved ones should be prepared to sign a contract with the funeral home and pay right then and there for the services to be provided. Be sure that the dollars involved are clear before signing anything, as those making the arrangements will be distraught and may be sorry later for contracting services not really wanted or needed.

If not already determined with your clergy, decisions will be made with the funeral director about the religious and/or funeral service;

coffin or cremation, and burial place; announcements in the newspaper and online guest books; and even the number of limousines. Many of these subjects are discussed in detail below. But it's always wise to have someone accompany whoever is making these choices – a child, close friend or possibly your clergy. Decide now who that should be and include it in your *Guide*.

Funeral Service

Practices, Policies, and Procedures
These vary not only, of course, from religion to religion, but also within a religion. They include what will or can happen at a funeral home, a house of worship, a cemetery, and at home. The best thing to do is to ask your clergy the possibilities "within his house." A funeral director (who conducts services for many religions), told me you can do anything you want, provided your clergy and children approve, except people are afraid to ask.

The Service

- Where will the service be held? And at what time?

- Who will officiate?

- Are there particular passages from the Bible, personal letters, poems, or anything else to be read?

- Is there favorite music to be played at the service?
  Any special instruments?

- Who will deliver the eulogy? Anything NOT to be said?
  Any limit on the number of speakers?

- Will there be an honor guard? Pall bearers?
  Who will notify them?

- Flowers? Who will arrange for them?

- Donations to a charity or charities need to be decided on
  now as this information could be included in a leaflet that

may be handed out at the funeral service, as well as printed in the newspaper.
(There is further discussion below about the obituary.)

Who will stay in your house during the service? The newspaper article will announce to one and all exactly when your house will be empty – even if the address is not shown in the newspaper - so have someone there to ward off an intruder.

Coffin, Burial Plots, and the Cemetery Service

Coffin

What kind of a coffin should be used? Any special requests as to the kind of material it should be made of or markings on it? Is there a preference if it is opened for viewing or should it be closed at all times?

Plots

Are cemetery plots paid for, and if so, where are they located? Are there deeds and where are they? Does your clergy or his house of worship know about the plots? If you don't own one, where do you want the burial to be?

Cemetery Service

If you counsel with your clergy in advance, you can state in your *Guide* what will happen at the cemetery to be sure it's what you want.

If you are Jewish, you may have special soil you want sprinkled on your casket. My wife and I have some earth from the Negev desert in Israel that is meaningful to us. Anything like that for you?

And mourners may be asked to shovel spades of earth onto the casket, as seems to be the custom today. Is this okay?

If the disposition of the body or cremated remains is not local, where is it? And who is the contact there? Clergy? Funeral director? Cemetery officials? Again, addresses and phone numbers should be shown.

Cremation
If this is desired, there are many questions:

- Does your religion allow it? And if not, do it anyway?

- Who will arrange the cremation?

- Who will perform the cremation? Would you like a special container?

- When will it be done in relation to any planned service?

- Who will retain the remains or ashes? Do you want to stipulate a meaningful place to spread the ashes?

Find out now who will help your survivors carry out your wishes. Your clergy or funeral director may be the ones to assist.

Like so many other issues, preferences must be known in advance and should be stated in your *Guide* so that your partner and/or executor will know what you want.

Reception After the Funeral
Once services are over, whether it is in a house of worship or at the cemetery, will guests be invited back for a light meal and beverage? How will people know? If so, who is making the arrangements, who is paying for it and where will it be?

Calling Hours
This will be decided in your conversation with clergy or the funeral director. Where will it be held? For how many days? And during which hours? Which members of the family should be there? Questions, questions, questions: easier to answer now when you can, rather than later when shock and grief are fresh.

The Obituary
An up-to-date resume (or curriculum vitae) is most helpful in writing an obituary, so it would be a good idea to include them for both partners in this section of your *Guide*. You don't want your surviving spouse to fumble around when your death is new, trying to remember

your educational background and achievements.

Resumes should include the following information with dates:

- Education

- Professional training

- Work history

- Service in the community

- Special careers

- Memberships in business and professional organizations, including offices held

- Publications and awards

- Personal information, which may include date of birth, marriage, divorce (if applicable), names of spouse, children and their spouses and offspring. Is there a former spouse or companion that should be mentioned?

Newspaper Article(s)

Your *Guide* should state:

- Who will write the article(s)

- Who should see it before submission

- Which newspapers to publish in

- How many days you would like the notice to appear

Are there organizations to notify? Your alumni association(s)? Religious organizations other than your own? Charitable organizations you gave time (and probably money) to?

Recently, newspapers, with their economic problems, are charging for notices and articles, so you will need to be mindful of the cost. Ask! Photograph: What picture, if any, would you like used? Where is it?

Charitable Contributions

Your friends may want to honor you with a contribution to a non-profit organization, so decide which one or ones you prefer. And while you are at it, what is the address of the agency? If there is more than one organization, what order do you want them listed in the paper? And is there a special fund within that charity you wish the money to go to?

The Death Certificate

Information that may be requested to complete the death certificate includes:

- Birthplace

- Father's and mother's names and birthplaces

- Social security number

- Usual occupation

Obtain from the funeral director or either state or city office, 15 copies with a raised seal for use later with governmental and insurance agencies.

There are so many questions. When do you want them answered? Now, when you both are able to discuss the answers – or later when your partner or loved ones will use his/her best judgment and hope it's the right answer?

Your call.

CHAPTER 6

Essential Contact Information

Yes, I'm a nut about being organized. I like to be able to retrieve information quickly and without a lot of hassle. I know the people I call to handle our finances and run the house. So why not list them for my partner and our executrix?

List here, as a ready reference for your loved ones, the names and contact information for people likely to be needed to settle your estate and to help your partner "Keep on Living." There might be two lists, as information may be different for you and your partner.

Contact information should include:

- The person's name

- His or her function

- The name of his or her assistant

- Name of the company/agency

- Location

- Telephone number

And the people needed to be called:

- Accountant

- Attorney

- Banker

- Credit card company

- Employer

- Insurance: – auto
                – life
                – dental
                – Long-Term Disability
                – medical for supplemental health care
                – prescription drugs

- Investment advisor

- Physician

- Social Security Department

CHAPTER 7

To Do Shortly After the Passing of a Loved One

Since I've taken care of certain family responsibilities over the years, I have come to understand the variety of tasks this entails. For example, being sure there's a sufficient cash balance in both my and my wife's checking accounts, managing investments, handling repairs to appliances, and making travel arrangements, including using miles for free tickets.

It's easy for me because I've done it. Now remove the anxiety for your partner and executor by recording what you know. This chapter will help you remember and educate your partner as to when to enlist the help of an advisor.

Engaging Your Professionals

Your surviving spouse or executor will need the assistance of professionals to help with the myriad of questions and *fears*. If these advisors are already chosen, don't be afraid to state in your *Guide* whom you trust (and especially those you might be a bit wary of).

But if advisors need to be chosen, there's a super piece online by Timberchase Financial. Page 8 of the article suggests good questions you can ask when interviewing these professionals. The article can be read by Googling: "Timberchase Financial What Do I Do Now."

Another article, in the *Wall Street Journal,* discusses these points and can be read by Googling: "How to Build Your Financial Dream Team," by Karen Blumenthal.

In either case, as with the funeral home, <u>it's always wise to have some-one accompany you – especially if you are speaking with someone new.</u> Certain tasks – i.e., the filing of IRS forms - can be performed by both your attorney and accountant, *so your partner and/or executor should find out in advance what each will do and the cost.* And unless there is total faith, get it in writing. This also avoids (secondary) af-ter shock. Although listed previously (in Chapter 6), recording them here with a telephone number, and if appropriate, account numbers, will make it easier. Include in your chart some of the functions these professionals perform, such as:

- <u>Attorney</u> – reviews your will and any trusts and makes certain the actions you wanted to happen really do. He or she is the one who will guide your estate through probate court, if necessary. That's the official place which transfers legal title from your estate to your designated beneficiaries.

And there is a relatively new field of law called Elder Law that ad-dresses issues facing seniors: estate planning, health care, retirement, taxes, abuse, and discrimination issues. In some states an attorney may be certified by The National Elder Law Foundation:

www.nelf.org

More information may be obtained at the website of The National Academy of Elder Law Attorneys, Inc.:

www.naela.com

For additional information, reach The Social Security and Disability Resource Center at:

www.ssdrc.com

- <u>Accountant</u> – assists your surviving spouse in determining where income will come from as well as helps list your assets and liabilities. This advisor should double check that all taxes have been paid and could make the calls to Social Security, the Veterans Administration, and other organizations.

- <u>Insurance Agent</u> for:

Auto Insurance	changes the name of the insured, if necessary, or will add names of children or grandchildren who will be driving your car(s).
Life Insurance	files the necessary paperwork so your loved ones receive the proceeds from your insurance policies; will also check that beneficiaries are updated.
Long Term Care Insurance	if applicable, helps survivors receive the monies to which they are entitled – even for those last hectic days.
Homeowners Insurance	verifies that the policy reads correctly and stays in force while assets are being transferred from your name to that of your surviving spouse.

- <u>Investment/Financial advisor</u> – determines, with your loved ones and your accountant, monthly or quarterly cash needs and helps to assess tolerance for risk in your investments. A single spouse may have less risk tolerance, so a change may be warranted in asset allocation (the percentage of the portfolio invested in stocks versus bonds). The advisor will additionally update your IRA beneficiaries. And if you visit with your investment advisor now, on a periodic basis, does your partner accompany you, to become as knowledgeable as possible?

If I were the surviving partner, I'd gather all the professionals in one room to decide who will do what and create a plan to avoid duplication and delay.

Moving Cash into the Checkbook

It's important for your partner to have an immediate sense of financial security, whether before or after contacting your professionals. There are several actions you can suggest so that financial self-confidence is achieved quickly:

- First, share how to determine the balance in each checking account, but state, as well, an approximate range of how much is normally kept in each account. Since these numbers constantly change, you must relate where that information is maintained. Be specific, and since this is so important, I'll tell you what my *Guide* says:

You can check the balance of both checkbooks by looking in the white notebook labeled "A & Z Checkbooks," which can be found in my office.

Specifically, you will find the notebook directly over my computer screen on the middle shelf.

In that notebook, and after the "ABC Register[3]" tab, you will find my check register (or for yours, after the "XYZ Register" tab). These pages show the current balance in each checking account.

- State how to transfer cash NOW from your checking account into that of your partner. Can't do it because each account is in one name only? Now is the time to put both names on each account, so your surviving partner is able to transfer money quickly in one of two ways:

  Using your checks (even though the check may have only your name on it), your partner can write one, made payable to him or herself and then deposit the check in the account that needs the cash.

  Or:

  If your survivor wishes, a transfer from your account to his or hers can be made easily either online, over the phone, or by going to the bank. Be sure to record the telephone number to call and where the pin number is located.

These options to access money immediately work because the accounts are in both names.

In either case, a small balance should be left in *your* account in case a check was written, not recorded in the check register, and then comes due for payment.

- Detail what to do when funds are needed in your partner's checkbook, but the cash in both her and your checking accounts has been spent. Whom to call? What information will be needed to transfer money from your investments into your spouse's checking account? (For ongoing access to cash, see Chapter 9.)

---

3. A "register" is a listing of checks.

Agencies to Notify

The following organizations need to be advised of your partner's new status:

- The Social Security Administration (800-772-1213) - so that your survivor can receive the death benefit and the higher of your two pensions (if one of your professional advisors hasn't already done so) – especially if your monthly payment is deposited automatically into your checking account.

- And be sure Medicare is contacted (800-633-4227) - to determine if there are any other benefits.

- If appropriate, call The Department of Veterans Affairs (800-827-1000) - for any military benefits.

- If you have two cars in the family, and a child or grandchild is (even temporarily) driving the extra car, be sure the insurance company is notified.

Cancellations

Plans have been made, insurance purchased and credit cards used. Unfortunately, all this must be changed and possibly canceled. Consider:

- How do your loved ones cancel your health insurance? Do you have double coverage – meaning that in addition to Medicare, you pay to cover the gap between what Medicare pays and what is charged (Medigap insurance)? Who needs to be called to cancel your insurance, but not that of your partner? What are the account and telephone numbers? Dental, prescription drug, life, and long term care insurance are in this category as well. So this one task could involve many calls, requiring significant amounts of information. Make a chart now because you know what to do.

- What social and travel plans have been made? Airlines? Hotels? Cruises? How were these reservations made? How can they be canceled so as not to waste precious money? Are there receipts or reservation forms anywhere in the house?

- What credit cards are in your name only? Where, physically, are the cards? Again, whom to call to cancel? What are the account and telephone numbers? This is important as it will stop any yearly automatic renewals of subscriptions to magazines, computer support programs, etc.

- Your driver's license will have to be canceled, so note the telephone number of the Department of Motor Vehicles in your state, and relay where your license is located.

- Online accounts to discontinue: Facebook (requires a death certificate to delete), Twitter, YouTube or others.

- Email accounts (i.e., gmail, yahoo, etc.) to close.

- Domain names for websites which will no longer be used.

Transfers

Transferring an account name is as important as canceling one. Which credit cards are in joint names that now need to be in one name? Whom to call? You should list the name of the credit card, the bank that issued it and the account and telephone numbers.

How about leases? Are any leases in your name only which do not end with your death – like your leased auto – that must be transferred to your survivor? How about your cell phone? Where is the paperwork?

Do you have unused airline miles? If transferable – and many are - these could come in handy if your partner decides to "get away" before having to face the ordeal of settling an estate.

Do you have membership in a club – eating or recreational – that could or should be transferred to your survivor's name?

What other information is in your head that will facilitate cancellations or transfers?

Automatic Charges

In this day of technology, there may be automatic monthly, quarterly or yearly charges to either a credit card or checking account. Consider payments charged to your:

- Credit card(s) that should be continued and therefore your survivor must tell the company to change the name on the card(s)

- Credit card(s) that should NOT be continued, to stop automatic renewals for things you no longer need or want

- Checking account(s) that should be continued and must be changed to your partner's name

- Checking account(s) that should be closed. It's important to know which payments are automatically charged to this/these accounts as they will stop. Are the payments for services you will still be using? If so, they'll need to be switched to the surviving partner's checking account

   Creating four charts for this information will clarify the status of these credit cards and checking accounts. Each should state the company, its phone number, account number, and what the charge is for.

Consider categories of companies that supply goods or services likely to be automatically deducted from your accounts:

- Airline, hotel, E-Z Pass, and rental car companies

- Computer support services – especially for software

- Health insurance providers

- Home maintenance such as burglar alarm or telephone or utility bills

- Newspaper subscriptions

- Places where you (frequently) purchase merchandise or books

- Your Internet service provider

To find additional companies you've dealt with, review your monthly banking and credit card statements <u>for the past year.</u>

Similarly, if you have set up bill-paying services through your bank, make sure these bills will be paid through your surviving partner's checking account.

Summary of Changes

For each account, plan or membership that needs to be canceled or transferred:

- Where is the actual card or paperwork located?

- Who should be called to make the change?

- What are the account and telephone numbers?

Tips for Living Alone

A couple of friends, Natalie Pelavin and Barbara Sosnowitz, PhD, have published a booklet entitled, *If We Knew Then What We Know Now*. This may be the first time your partner is living alone for a prolonged period and may not feel safe. Here are some of Natalie's and Barbara's pointers to relieve that anxiety:

- Keep a cell phone in its charger on a nightstand. If landline service is interrupted, there will be a way to communicate.

- Know where flashlights are kept that work. Keep extra batteries on hand. Consider buying a flashlight that plugs into the wall, which will always be charged and which will shine a small light when the power goes off.

- Many single people change their telephone directory listing to include initials only – for an added bit of anonymity.

- Know that 911 paramedics will break down the door if the person inside can't get to the door to open it.

- Have your loved ones learn how to use the house alarm system. (See Chapter 17.)

- Your partner may want to change the house key and the alarm code, and then distribute a list of those to people who have access to your home. (Also see Chapter 17.)

And if you want to order this booklet, email NPelavin@yahoo.com for your own copy.

Medical Alert System
Now that your partner will be living alone, might it be wise to have a medical alert device in case of an emergency? In addition, it could give your children and grandchildren a sense of comfort.

Pets
Taking future care of your pet(s) should be high on your list. What becomes of him/her/them if something unexpected happens to you? Possibly you have established a trust for future care, as many states now allow, or your local SPCA can be involved. In addition, some Schools of Veterinary Medicine will assume responsibility for the pet if you have created an endowment at the school.

A New Will or Trust
Your survivor will need to place on a "To Do" list a discussion with your attorney whether or not a new will and/or trust are needed. Any new Powers of Attorney required?

Memorial Plaque in Your House of Worship
Many houses of worship have memorial plaques to remember departed members of the congregation. Do you want one with your name on it? If so, who should be contacted?

Head or Tombstone
Would you like to request special markings that you want on these stones? Who will know if you don't write them down and tell others?

CHAPTER 8

Information You'll Need Later

Not everything can be done at once – especially after the loss of a loved one - but I know there will be certain pieces of information that need to be accessed easily so that my wife can live well, or so our executor can settle the estate. I've listed them for my survivors and think you should too.

Legal Papers

Wills and Trusts

A will is a legal document by which a person designates a survivor (called an "executor" or "executrix") to manage the affairs of the estate. A will, moreover, also provides for the transfer of property.

A **trust** is also a legal document which establishes a relationship so that property is held by one party (called the "trustee") for the benefit of a second party.

Be sure your survivors know where these documents are located; state the name and telephone number of the attorney who prepared them – if there was one.

It will be meaningful to describe the contents and purpose of these documents as if you were talking to the survivor. Why did you make these provisions? Any special instructions for your loved ones? Use plain English; remember, no one will see these instructions except your partner, estate attorney and executor, so be clear. This is your opportunity to establish what you want to accomplish after you pass.

Property Distribution Lists

These are documents that tell your partner and/or executor of your estate what to do with certain pieces of property. Do you have a favorite chair or piece of jewelry or heirloom that you want to be sure is given to a specific person?

And be sure to let your loved ones know where these property lists are.

Types of Lists

- <u>Memo of Distribution.</u> My wife and I created this easily by copying our Valuable Items insurance policy and designated, in our handwriting, beneficiaries of particular pieces. We signed each page and gave it to our estate attorney.

- <u>Specific Asset Distribution.</u> An example: Your entire estate is divided equally among your children, except that you want to leave a particular piece of property (real estate, a business, etc.), to certain children. This is where you could state that. Another example could be an investment account that was inherited by one of you (in a previous marriage), that you want left to only the children of the inheritor.

Either of these documents may or may not be part of your will – depending upon the advice of your attorney. What's important is that your wishes be in writing and carried out upon your death.

Other Papers
These could include certificates of birth, marriage, divorce, military service and death. But where are they? Be sure to note their location.

Are there any other important documents? Do you have ownership in a going business? If so, how would <u>you</u> go about evaluating your interest? How will your loved ones determine unpaid salary, commission or royalties? Do you have any other continuing income? Be sure your loved ones know about it.

<u>Evaluations for the Estate</u>

Appraisals
Are there any jewelry, art, or business appraisals that would be of value to your partner or estate? If so, be sure to describe them and state the exact location.

Collections/Hobbies

Do you have any collections that are of value? Do you know where to have them appraised or possibly sold after your death? Is there an inventory of what you have? This category is unlimited but could include classical CDs, Russian boxes, silver miniatures, etc., etc. One person I know has a wonderful assortment of walking sticks and canes, another collects scissors. What have you accumulated along the way? And to whom should it be given or sold?

Taking photographs of collectibles, antiques and antique furniture, paintings and decorative items might be a good idea, as photos are often helpful if collections are sold later.

(By the way, if there will be many people in the house after the funeral, there might be someone with sticky fingers! Pictures will be helpful to your insurance company, in case of loss.)

Other

Safe Deposit Box

If you have one, what's in it? And where is the box located? Where are the keys? Is the rental on automatic renewal? If so, to which credit card or bank account is the rental charged? And later, will you need the box at all?

So many questions – all of which will have to be answered - either by you now, because you took the time, or by your survivors later, who may or may not handle arrangements and issues as you may want. And if it's left up to your survivors, it could very well be the basis for disputes or at least hard feelings.

So take the time. Do it now, and know that you will still be doing your part to promote harmonious family relationships.

Section 2
Part B
Information So Your Loved Ones
Can Go On Living

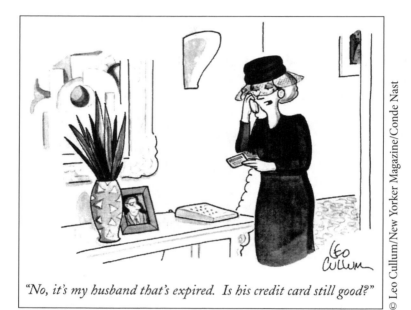

CHAPTER 9

Financial Information (Banking and Bills)

I've worked hard to provide a high standard of living for my family. When I retired, it was important to me that our lives maintain the quality enjoyed when I ran a business. But I know that my memory is not my best asset, so I've had to be organized. Since I want my wife to keep on living well after I'm gone (and also want our estate plan carried out properly), I have felt compelled to write down information housed only in my mind, so others can know it. One of the most important areas of knowledge to pass on, of course, concerns our finances.

Again, a word of caution: much of the information you must relate is highly personal, and you don't want account numbers floating around. So the location of these facts – either in your *Guide* or referenced there - must be secure!

Sources of Income and Assets, and Debts

In General
For each item of income due or monies owed by you, be sure to state:

- Each person or entity from whom money is coming, and everyone who needs to be paid

- Any account numbers for identification

- The location of supporting documents

- Why it is due or payable – details that explain the particular financial arrangement

And, in addition, for any asset, describe what it is and your percentage of ownership.

Why Is This Important to Know? Because your:

Income	will determine your partner's standard of living and future lifestyle.
Assets	will tell him or her where the income comes from.
Debts	will state how much you owe and to whom, which will impact what your partner will be able to afford and need to budget for in the future.

Income

List income from all sources, so your surviving spouse doesn't have to seek it out and most importantly, doesn't miss anything.

Sources of income can include:

- Salary that is still due

- Monthly Social Security payments

- Investments

- Property on consignment, which when sold will yield income

- Business partnership residuals

- Rental or timeshare properties you own

- Deposits to be returned – for example, from a proposed move to a retirement home or cancelled trips

- Tax rebates

- Royalties or residuals from a business, books, or music

- Life insurance proceeds

- Pensions or annuities

- Monies due from others (loans or mortgages granted)

Be sure to state what income, if any, is received automatically – that is, deposited directly into your checking account or that of your surviving spouse.

Assets

Assets are defined as something you own, which can produce money in your pocket, such as:

- Checking or savings accounts

- Real estate

- Business ownership

- Pending contracts that could produce income in the future

- Automobiles and boats (if leased, see Chapter 12)

- Tangible personal property (anything you own that's moveable), such as jewelry, furniture or artwork

- Cash or traveler's checks kept in the house

- Unredeemed miles from an airline that can be turned into cash

Digital Assets

We all know about material assets, as described in the previous list, but with the advent of technology, there are digital assets. These have cash value or may have to be canceled:

- Online rebates for past purchases (big box office supply companies come to mind)

- Items listed on eBay or Craigslist

- PayPal accounts which may have monies that can be drawn out or an amount due to a third party

Debts

Equally important are your debts. For instance:

- Credit card balances

- Unpaid mortgage(s) and home equity lines of credit

- Unpaid bills

- City, state or federal taxes

- Student loans

- Personal or business loans

Again, are bills paid or are payments automatically deducted from a checking account or charged to a credit card? Which card? For car leases? Utility bills? Mortgage? Health insurance? Cell phone?

<u>Checkbooks</u>

For <u>each checkbook</u>, you need to state:

- The bank's name and the checkbook number

- The purpose of the account
  (Is it a joint account, and if not, why?)

- Who can sign checks on this account
  (My wife and I maintain separate accounts and while each
  check shows only one name, each of us can sign the other's
  checks. Thus, neither of us will have a delay in accessing the
  balance of the other.)

- Where you keep the checks, checkbook, and current or
  past statements
  (Is it balanced monthly?)

- How you maintain the register (the listing of checks written)
  Manually? On the computer?
  (And where is the register?)

- If there are any recently closed accounts that you want your survivors to know about

- Any abbreviations that are obvious only to you
  (I use "TY" and "LY" for "this year" and "last year" and "TM" and "LM" for "this month" and "last month.")

Your partner should ask your professionals how long to keep your checkbook open (with a minimum balance) in case there is a refund from the IRS or life insurance premium, to make sure all checks written on the account have cleared, or if a check wasn't entered properly in your register.

Access to Cash - Ongoing

Since your surviving spouse has had you, the financial manager, to replenish the checkbook with cash, this could be a daunting task, so be specific.

How is money transferred into your partner's bank checkbook once the balances in both checkbooks are spent? Is there someone to call? And what exactly does that person do?

Possibly, you have several investment accounts, each with its own checkbook. And you may know how to go online to determine which investment account has an available cash balance – so you won't write a check that will bounce. You know to merely deposit that check from your investment account into your bank checkbook. Easy for you. But not for someone who has not done it.

So you must explain exactly what to do.

My *Guide* says this:

"To obtain cash, call Ms. X and Mr. Y (the names of our investment/ financial advisor and that of her assistant) at 401-xxx-xxxx, who will determine which investment account to write the check from, and who will make sure the (name of investment company) check you write will not bounce. Should this drain the account of cash, Ms. X will replenish the account by selling securities or bonds to create cash.

"Or, you can ask them to transfer this cash directly into your checking account (number and name of bank).

"I was always sure I had no less than a $xx,xxx cash balance in either my investment account, #AAA or yours, #BBB, both of which have checkbooks, which are found in (state location)."
(Learn to identify locations in Chapters 25 -27.)

ATM Cards
This is yet another way of obtaining cash. How many cards are there? Where are they? For each card, what is the pin number to withdraw cash at the ATM – a/k/a "the money wall"? Where are these pin numbers written down? Is there a limit to the amount of cash you can obtain at any one time?

Credit Cards
For each credit card, your survivors should know:

- The bank that issued the card, its number and the credit limit

- That each card has a 3 or 4 digit verification code, also called a CVV or security or identification code, located on the back of the card, which may be required when ordering merchandise online

- What you use this card for

- Whom you call to cancel the card
  (This will immediately stop any automatic renewals of computer software, dining discount cards or magazine subscriptions, etc., as well as the card itself.)

It is a good idea to photocopy both sides of your credit cards, but then note in your *Guide* where these copies can be found. Be sure it's a secure place.

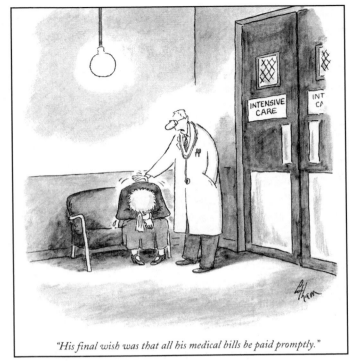

"His final wish was that all his medical bills be paid promptly."

Unpaid Bills

Where are these kept? Does that location include bills issued once a year, that have (unpaid) quarterly payments, such as those related to taxes? How will your surviving spouse know partial payments have been made?

Paid Bills

Almost as important as unpaid bills are the paid ones, as these may be necessary for your surviving spouse to do your taxes. Do paid bills show the date paid, check number and amount? If not, how will she know that they have been paid so they are not paid twice?

And where are they kept? (Look ahead to Chapter 25, "How to Identify Locations of Documents.")

Home Mortgages

Maybe by this time you don't have a mortgage, but if you do, does your information include:

- The name of the institution issuing the mortgage and the property that is mortgaged?

- The due date and amount of the payment? When the mortgage ends?

- Knowledge that paying more than the minimum due will decrease the amount of interest paid and will reduce the time it will take to pay it off?

- The location of the mortgage documents?

Taxes
There are income taxes and property taxes, so let's take each separately.

Income Taxes
There may be a great deal of information in your head on this subject, and it may be recorded under "Unpaid Bills" in the paragraph above, but your surviving spouse needs to know:

- That there are quarterly tax payments due for both federal and state (and maybe city or county) governments and the location of coupons to be mailed with each payment (which state amount and due date). How will he or she know which taxes have already been paid?

- How you go about gathering the information for your taxes. (See "Income and Expenses" paragraph below.)

- Where the information is kept so your survivors can give it to your accountant for the coming year.

- Who prepares and files your taxes. If you did your own tax preparation and filing, what do you suggest for your surviving spouse, and who will do this task in the future?

- Any special situations, such as losses in the past, which your accountant should be informed of.

Property Taxes

Again, you may have stated everything there is to know about these taxes in the "Unpaid Bills" paragraph, but if not, then what is your advice?

Tax Returns

These documents get special mention because they are so important. Be sure your survivor and/or executor know where past returns are located. (See Chapter 27, "Locations of Specific Documents.")

Income and Expenses

Do you keep track of your income and expenses for tax or budgetary purposes? Let your loved ones know your record keeping and information gathering procedures and where they are located. For example, do you use an online program or ledger system?

If you don't use a computer program that tracks income and expenses, maybe you should consider it. A summary of how your money has been spent for the past few years will give your survivor a road map to a future standard of living and assist with maintaining or altering a budget.

If you wanted, you could go a step further and prepare a summary of what future income will be (without any income attributable to you) and future expenses (again without items pertaining to you).

Handling Finances in the Future

What advice do you have for:

- Paying taxes and bills? Should someone be engaged to do this to reduce stress? If so, how to find someone? Your attorney, accountant or wealth advisor (all of whom have been through this before) may know of people who will come to the house. Certainly friends in the same position can recommend someone to be interviewed.

- Managing large sums of money that may be received from life insurance proceeds, final payouts from pension funds or even proceeds from inheritance, etc?

- Making irreversible financial decisions like selling property, downsizing, or giving away life insurance proceeds?

- And, although stated before, but it bears repeating: <u>Whom do you trust and of whom should your survivors be a bit wary?</u>

<u>Document Disposal and Shredding</u>
Part of gaining control of your finances is knowing not only where documents are but also when to dispose of them – if ever.

But how long should receipts, bills and paperwork be kept? This depends on what it is, and in many cases, whom you ask. To make matters simple, Appendix A lists documents and when to dispose of them.

And speaking of disposal, you should shred anything you don't need to keep. If you purchase your own shredder, be sure it's a "cross-cut" one. Otherwise the machine will cut papers into long bands which could be pieced back together.

In addition, you can use the Internet to find a community shredding event – sometimes in a police station or shopping center parking lot – and these are usually free. Another choice is to take your documents to a company who will do it for you, and there are those who will come to your home to do the shredding.

CHAPTER 10

Investments

Investments and investment accounts can be complicated – assets all over the place. In our case they are simple, or so I think. Because they may seem involved to others, I have been careful to explain them in the Guide I have left for my wife and survivors – especially accounts that are "off to the side" and not professionally managed.

The information for accounts includes what the investment is, where it is, why we have our investments in the form we do and whom to contact. It's my way of showing love and trying to continue to protect my wife, children and grandchildren. I know you feel the same.

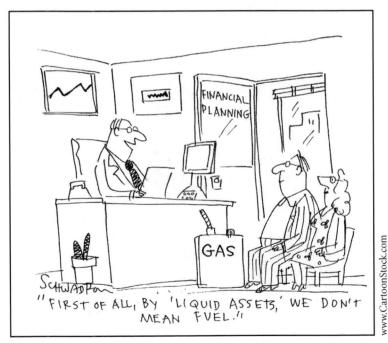

"FIRST OF ALL, BY 'LIQUID ASSETS,' WE DON'T MEAN FUEL."

Discuss These Issues Now!

Many decisions can be made by both your partner and you before your death. Likewise, the time to teach your survivor about your investments is now. If you visit with your advisor periodically, be sure that you both are present.

Investment Advisor or Broker

One of the first people to be contacted by your partner, in addition to your attorney, should be your investment or wealth advisor or your broker representative, if you have one. Your professionals will help your surviving spouse understand his or her financial condition. (Telephone numbers are listed in Chapter 6.)

If you don't have a professional advisor, whom should your surviving spouse contact about your account(s)? Now is the time to say – don't make her or him guess later!

- What were your reasons for your choice of this person or firm? Is there one special person whom you trust and have faith in, or was it the company?

- Your investment advisor, especially if it's a bank, may perform services other than managing your investments, such as paying bills or taxes. And they could be at no charge – so be sure you ask and advise your survivor!

Investment Advisor Agreement

If you have a professional advisor, you may have an agreement with him, her or the firm, and it is important to explain to your surviving spouse the important parts of this document.

- How much are you paying for these services? How are they paid? If the principle decreases below a certain point, does the fee increase?

- Explain that there are different ways to pay your financial advisors including: an asset-based fee, fee plus commissions, a flat fee, a percentage of net worth and income, or by the hour.

  These are discussed in a *Wall Street Journal* article by Daisy Maxey. Google: "How to Pay Your Investment Advisor."

- Can the advisor be replaced if your survivors are not pleased?

Investment Accounts

There is a great deal of information about your investment accounts that you can impart so your surviving spouse will be more knowledgeable when speaking with your professional.

Here are some suggestions on information to share:

- What is/are the account number(s) and which bank or brokerage house ("the custodian") holds the assets?

- What type of account is it - (IRA, Roth IRA, trust, a simple investment account, etc.)? In whose name is each account? What happens to those accounts currently in your name?

- What is the purpose of each account? Why aren't all the accounts rolled into one? Describe the benefits or restrictions of each.

- Are there checkbooks attached to any of these accounts that your surviving spouse can use to access cash?

- How does your surviving spouse know if there's enough cash in the account to cover the check he or she is about to write? (See Chapter 9)

Investment Reports

When investment reports arrive, teach your partner how to read them; explain what they mean. This will also give her or him confidence to know what they're all about, rather than being one more area to decipher later.

Explain the difference between the two investment reports sent – one from your advisor, probably quarterly, and the second from the custodian (bank or brokerage company), probably monthly. What does your survivor do with them? How long should they be kept?

Why do you have the asset allocation that you do? What is asset allocation, anyway?

Your custodian may additionally send "tax information" reports during January or February to be used for the filing of last year's taxes. Explain what these do and what to do with them. (You <u>do</u> have lots of information in your head.)

Many investment questions can be answered:

- How is the yearly return determined? And on which report can this be found?

- What is a reasonable rate of return to expect? Are there any standards with which to compare your results?

- What period of time is realistic to evaluate investment results?

And you have the answers...or know who does!

Real Estate Investments
Possibly you own a second home, which you rent either on a seasonal or year-round basis. If so, there's information which must be passed on.

Current Rentals and Leases
First, where are the leases located and what are the terms? Who collects the rent and when do the leases end?

Financial Information
Do you own the property or do you have partners? Is there a mortgage? If so:

- To whom are payments made? What is the amount of the monthly payment?

- Where is the mortgage paperwork located?

- When does it end?

- In addition, do you tally the income and expenses at the end of the year to determine if the property is still worth owning? If so, where are those figures?

Insurance

Do you have a copy of the insurance policy on the property? From whom do you obtain it? How much does it cost each year?

Keys

Who has keys to the property? If you do, where are they?

Purchase and Improvements

Where are the closing papers? Is the deed to the property included in that file? Do you remember the professionals involved - the attorney and/or real estate broker? Do you or your accountant have a record of improvements made to the house over the years?

Property Manager Arrangements

If you have a property manager, who is it? Be sure to relate:

- Name and telephone number of person or company

- Term of management
  (When does the contract with him/her/them end?)

- How much their services cost
  (From which account is a check written?)

- Which services are provided
  (Who seeks new tenants? Is the rental agent different from the property manager?)

Property Maintenance

What is the manager's responsibility for maintenance? Weekly mowing and landscaping? Snow shoveling, if applicable? Any restrictions, such as how much can be spent for repairs before your OK is required?

Rented Equipment

If anything is rented – such as a hot water heater – who pays for it? What are the terms of the rental?

Other Investment Issues

Special Insights

You may have purchased an investment due to reasons known only to yourself, and these securities may be held in an account separate from other assets. This is the time and place to share your reasoning so your surviving spouse can realize the benefit. What event or price would have told you it is time to sell? Ever? Or should this investment be passed on to the children? And why?

Costs of Investments

Most of the time your advisor or custodian will know this, but possibly you have a "personal investment account" – which your advisor has no knowledge about or control over, as you're the one responsible for the investments. Where are the costs of these investments? Does your broker or custodian have them? Do you have a file that contains this information? Don't make people seek the hiding place for this information – it's too expensive!

Will the Money Last? A Life Projection

This is possibly one of the most important questions your surviving spouse will ask. When I first retired, my advisor opened my eyes with a simple explanation that was presented as a chart or spreadsheet.

"You are starting with x dollars, and yearly we can project they will earn a given percentage. That adds to the pot. And each year you will withdraw money to live on, and therefore, if this is done for the next so-many years, you will run out of money in such-in-such year."

Here's what a chart might look like:[4]

Year End	Start	Earn 5%	Withdraw	End
2013	$1000	$50	$40	$1010
2014	$1010	$51	$40	$1021
2015	$1021	$51	$40	$1032
2016	$1032	$52	$40	$1043
2017	$1043	$52	$40	$1055

4. The charts in this chapter are constructed more easily in a spreadsheet program, which is what I have used. All figures are rounded off.

Note that the starting balance, of course, equals the ending balance of the prior year. In this case the assumed earnings per year are 5% and the yearly projected withdrawal is a constant $40. Since you are earning more per year than you are taking out, the balance at the end of 5 years increases. However, if you earn less than you draw out (3% in the chart below), then the balance obviously diminishes. The chart will tell you when your nest egg will run out. Better yet, it will alert you in advance so withdrawals (spending) can be adjusted, assuming you can't do anything about the amount coming into the pot (earnings).

Year End	Start	Earn 3%	Withdraw	End
2013	$1000	$30	$40	$990
2014	$990	$30	$40	$980
2015	$980	$29	$40	$969
2016	$969	$29	$40	$958
2017	$958	$29	$40	$947

That simple chart was a shocker and even though digits usually talk to me, I just didn't think of it that way.

I call it a "Life Projection," and each year I compare the actual ending balance of all the accounts to the projected ending amount – what I thought the account balance would be at the end of that year. If we had less money than anticipated, I try to figure out why. Was the investment return below expectations, or are we spending too much? And this determines our lifestyle (that is, spending) so that not only will the money last, but there will be a certain amount of money left at the age I'm guessing we'll be when we both die.

But, naturally, there are many variables:

- What will be the rate of return on the investments?

- How much will be drawn out each year?

- How long does the money have to last?

- And should there be anything left when both your partner and you die?

Who will handle this most important function after you're gone?

That's why you need to make the effort to explain this – while you can – because your loved ones are worth it, and you want to do what you can now to protect and help them later – when you're not here.

CHAPTER 11

Insurance

Insurance policies – and many legal documents – seem to be written in a foreign language, so I rely on professionals. More than once, I have handed one of these documents back and simply commented, "What DOES this say?"

It's so easy to miss important aspects of insurance coverage, and that's why it's important to state in your own words what you know will be meaningful to your survivor. But don't be afraid to ask your insurance agent questions. I feel that the only really stupid question is the one that is not asked. You may be sure that yours has been asked before.

Information Common to All Policies

For many types of insurance, the information recorded is the same although there may be details pertinent to that particular coverage. Here are questions for you to answer that apply to most insurance policies:

- What is the name of the insurance company?

- What is the policy number?

- Whom do you call for questions on the policy? Telephone number?

- What type of insurance is this and what is it for?

- What or who is covered? Any restrictions or limitations?

- How much does it cost? And for what time period?

- How is it paid: by check upon receipt of a bill, deducted from your Social Security payment, or automatically charged to your credit card or checking account? If a bill will be received, from whom – the insurance company? The broker?

- Policy limit – what is the maximum that the insurance company will pay out?

- Whom do you call to submit a claim? Telephone number?

- How can it be canceled?

- Where is policy located?

- How often should your partner obtain quotations on the cost? This is especially true of supplemental or Medigap health insurance as well as Plan D drug insurance (both discussed below), as what's covered and what's not, changes not only from year to year but from one policy to another.

Are there provisions to policies, specific to that type of coverage, that need to be explained?

Automobile

- In case of an accident, what is the deductible (the amount of money the policy holder must pay before the insurance company pays)? To whom do you report an accident? Just the insurance agent – or the insurance company – or both? Are there any situations when you do not want to report it and just pay the damages?

- Do you have a recommended place to take the car to have it fixed? What's the name, address and phone number of the auto body shop? Is there someone special you deal with? Does your insurance include the rental of a loaner car? And what type of car are you entitled to?

Health Insurance

As we get older, medical insurance becomes more and more important, as, unfortunately, we undergo tests we didn't even know existed. So it's necessary to describe what health insurance plans you have. "Medicare" can consist of different parts:

- Part A is hospital insurance that helps cover inpatient care in hospitals, skilled nursing facilities, hospice, and at home. Part A also covers lab work and x-rays while in the hospital.

- Part B helps cover medically-necessary care, such as doctor's services, outpatient care, durable medical equipment, home health services, as well as outpatient lab work and x-rays.

- Plan C is a combination of Plans A, B (and sometimes) D issued by private companies approved by Medicare. It is also called a Medicare Advantage Plan.

- Plan D is for prescription drugs.

For further explanations to use in your *Guide*, Google: "Medicare Benefits provide details on Cost, Coverage," and scroll down to the article with that title.

Supplemental or Medigap Insurance

Plans A and B of Medicare pay for many medical bills but not everything, so privately purchased supplemental (called "Medigap") insurance will cover part or all of the difference between what is charged and what Medicare will pay. If you have a Medigap policy, is prior authorization from the insurance company or a second medical opinion required before your insurance company will pay the claim?

Plan D Drug Coverage

Unquestionably, this is difficult to explain as there are many types of plans, and each state has its own set of choices. Suffice it to say that you need to relate the provisions of what's in your plan:

- Whether a drug your family uses is covered at all, since each plan has its own list of drugs that it will pay for. The list of covered drugs is called a "formulary." Do you have a copy of yours? Where?

- The deductible – how much do you pay before the insurance company pays anything?

- The co-payment for each prescription.

When the "donut hole"[5] kicks in (if it's applicable to your plan), who pays how much after that?

Dental Insurance
Be sure you describe the limitations – both monetary and for types of service.

Homeowners

- What is the deductible? Is it appropriate for the coverage and premium?

- Are there specific conditions that are covered or exempted?

- Are you still covered if you renovate or vacate your home for more than 30 days?

- Is the amount of insurance on your home adequate to rebuild it?

- Is identity theft covered? Will your policy pay for forgery, counterfeit money, and losses from electronic fund transfers and credit cards?

- Do you put this coverage out to bid every three years? If so, how do you handle it?

---

5. Medicare drug plans may have a "coverage gap," which is sometimes called the "donut hole." This means that after you and your plan have spent a certain amount of money for covered drugs, you have to pay all costs out-of-pocket for your drugs (up to a limit). Your yearly deductible, coinsurance or copayments, and what you pay in the coverage gap all count toward this out-of-pocket limit. The limit doesn't include the drug plan's premium.

Life Insurance

- List the type of insurance: whole life or term?

- Who owns the policy? (Sometimes it is necessary to explain that the original insurance company was sold so there's one name on the policy and another one on the bill.)

- Who is insured?

- Who is the beneficiary?

Long Term Care Insurance

- What are the details of what the insurance company will pay? Does it increase each year? How does that work?

- Is there a waiting period before the benefit is paid?

- To determine what "triggers" a benefit, it's best to check with your insurance agent.

- To give your survivor some comfort, you may want to reference the Genworth Life Insurance Company's "Cost of Care Survey" by Googling: "Genworth Cost of Care for *your state*."

Personal Liability Insurance

- While this insurance covers you for a claim or suit against you for damages of bodily injury, personal injury or personal damage caused by an occurrence, are there situations NOT covered? How about if you operate a home day care business?

- Do you have Umbrella or excess liability insurance over and above your primary coverage?

Professional Insurance

If you have special coverage because of your occupation, such as professional liability or malpractice insurance, here is the place to tell your survivors about it. Doctors, attorneys, accountants and mediators, among others, have this kind of protection. How long does it need to remain in effect after your passing?

Valuable Items Insurance

- Are you insured for today's replacement cost or for a depreciated value?

- How long since this policy was updated? Do you still possess all the items or have you given away (or will you bequeath) pieces?

Other Miscellaneous Insurance

Renters
If you are renting property, be sure to include this coverage in your charts and explanations.

Travel Emergency
This is a special policy that provides you personal assistance when you are away from home and have a medical or travel emergency – regardless of where you are in the world. Since it's not expensive and fortunately not often used, your survivors may have forgotten about it. How about telling your children about it in case it's needed?

Water Line
Another special situation insurance, this provides coverage if the water pipe breaks between your street and your house. In our area, the water company is not financially responsible to fix it. Is it in yours?

Officers and Board of Directors Involvement
Are you covered by a for-profit or non-profit organization for your service as an officer or member of the board? It is true that good deeds may not go unpunished.

CHAPTER 12

Leases

Check the fine print in leases! You've heard it before: the devil is in the details, and I was astounded to learn that our car leases do not end with the death of the lessee. I was also taken in by cell phone insurance, which, for certain carriers, is a waste of money after 20 months. After that, if you were to lose your phone, you can get an upgraded new one for $50 or less. If you claim the loss against your insurance, there's a $50 deductible. It costs $50 either way, so why pay for insurance?

Automobile Leases

In addition to stating their location, you need to relate the following for each lease:

- The monthly rental cost

- Special features or protections included in the lease payment

- From whom the car is leased, and who sends the bill

- If property taxes are extra, and if so, how much they are, and who sends the bill

- What happens in case of death and if there is a death benefit

- When the lease ends

Cell Phones

Again, in addition to locating the original paperwork for your surviving spouse, the following could be helpful for each phone in the family:

- How much is the monthly rental?

- What does this cover? Number of minutes? Limited area? International?

- Who did you buy the phone contract from? And who sends the bill?

- Does the monthly rental include anything else, such as insurance, in case you lose or drop a phone? If so, is there a deductible?

- How does one file a claim if the phone is dropped or lost?

- Have you paid for support? Is there a number to call to learn how to use the phone? If so, how much does this cost? And when does this benefit end?

- What happens in case of death?

- When does the phone contract end?

Other Leases
Have you leased a house or a condo for the winter or summer? Where is that agreement? Are there any other leases to which you have agreed?

CHAPTER 13

Health and Medical

You know that the new bar scene for seniors is a doctor's office, and you also know you're a senior when more people want to see your health insurance cards in a given week than your VISA® or MasterCard®. As we age, health becomes more and more of an issue, so it's important that those around you know all about the people, medications and documents that help maintain your and your partner's good health.

Medical Alert System

As mentioned in Chapter 7, seniors living alone should consider having a medical alert system, as it provides a sense of security, not only to your partner, but also to your children and grandchildren.

Doctors

Your surviving partner probably knows your physicians, and once you are gone, it doesn't matter. But what if both your surviving spouse and/ or you are unable to communicate after an accident and your executor or executrix – possibly your child – needs to know this information?

A list is easy to make and it should show:

- Name of physician or surgeon

- Who uses this doctor – your spouse or you?

- Address and telephone number

- Medical specialty

Medications

Sure, your spouse may know what you take, but how about your executor or executrix? For this third person, your list should include:

- The name and strength of the medication

- Who is taking it

- How often it is taken

- Who prescribed it and for what purpose

- Where refills are obtained

Possibly you buy some of your medications outside the United States. If so, which one(s), from whom and at what cost? How do you reorder – by telephone or online? And where is the paperwork from prior order(s)?

Insurance

This subject is covered in detail in Chapter 11.

Insurance Cards - Health and Dental

Have you made copies of these cards? It saves a lot of number copying, as the first thing a health provider wants, of course, is a copy of your insurance card. This is a good place to let your surviving spouse know where these copies are.

Other Medical Information

It is prudent to discuss with your legal professional whether you should have the three legal documents described below. If you do, list them in a chart that shows the name of the document, who prepared it, who has copies, the location of your copy, and a brief description of what it says – in your words, as legalese is sometimes difficult to understand.

Durable Power of Attorney – Health

This gives the power to make health decisions on your behalf to another person (each other or a third person) in case you are incapacitated.

A Living Will
A legal document stating the kinds of treatments you want and do not want; it does not choose a specific person to carry out your wishes, which is accomplished in the Durable Power of Attorney – Health.

Durable Power of Attorney to Use Health Information
This allows your health care providers to release your medical information so that proper care may be given. It may be another item for the chart.

The following information needs to be included in your *Guide* as well:

Eyeglass Prescription
I'm sure you have a spare pair, so detail where it is, the name of the doctor who prescribed it and the optometrist who supplied the glasses.

Medical Records
Is there some file in which you keep old blood pressure, lab, or other medical reports?

My past reports came in mighty handy when my doctor noticed results that seemed "out of range." It turned out that, because I had the data from a few years past, these readings were always "out of range," and it was concluded that my "normal" is different from the standard, and no further observation was necessary.

CHAPTER 14

Charitable Giving

My wife and I have spent most of our lives helping others – not only with charitable contributions, but more importantly, with our time, effort and any talents we may have. But money is important! So it is only natural that I want our charitable efforts to continue to improve life for others. Maybe you feel the same way. And if you do, you need to include this information in your Guide.

Unpaid Pledges

Here's another bit of your life you may be carrying around in your head. Oh! Yes, it's all written down somewhere – but that won't help your loved ones if no one else knows where. So let's start with a chart of what you have pledged but not paid. The chart could include:

- Date of the original commitment

- Organization receiving the pledge

- What it is for (capital campaign, yearly dues or annual giving - and if a multi-year pledge)

- Amount of the total commitment

- How much was paid and when

- When the recipient expects to be paid: yearly or quarterly

- The amount of each payment

- Date the next payment should be made

As is true of everything else, where are documents or pledges located?

How Pledges Are Paid
As important as knowing what is to be paid and for how long, your survivors need to understand where the money comes from to make the payments.

Your sources could be:

- Your checkbook – out of ordinary income
  Give your surviving spouse an idea of what you've spent the past few years by reviewing your federal or state income tax returns.

- Funds or pools of money that you've established at a local charity or foundation.

  If you have set up pledges to be paid from this type of fund, you need to provide details on where each is located, who has authority over it, whom to contact, how to authorize the charity to make payments – and generally how it works. You may want to explain your reasoning for establishing the fund where you did, so survivors can honor your choice if it has special meaning for you.

  What happens to the fund after your survivors die?

Your professional advisors will probably be able to provide considerable support in this area.

History of Giving
Have you ever constructed a chart showing all of your charitable giving, including the sources for payments and the various recipients? If so, it would give your surviving spouse an idea of how much in total was donated and how you have been making payments.

Oftentimes a charity will call and say, "Last year..." A history would be most valuable in answering these calls for monetary donations, since it would relate what you've done in the past and allow him or her to continue what the two of you did together. Likewise, if the amount needs to be reduced, it could assist your partner in making that decision.

CHAPTER 15

Home Service Repairs and Maintenance

The other day, our dryer wouldn't work. No amount of button pushing or even a call to their national service center helped. It took a costly service visit to learn which two buttons to push together. I wish I had remembered to look in my wife's Guide which stated how to fix the problem!

We also have a whirlpool bathtub with a mind of its own. Ten minutes after you shut it off, it goes on again. Frankly, I push the "off" button a few times since it's too big to throw out the window, and it seems to work, but my wife thinks I have a magic touch.

OK, this is one of my responsibilities in our relationship. Our home is our fortress – protection from the outside – but it takes a great deal of effort (and a little common sense) to live comfortably, and I want that to continue when I'm not here. It was this need to have the house run smoothly without me that prompted me to include this information. It should be available for your loved ones, too.

Which Repair/Maintenance Professionals to List:

- Air Conditioning (and Heating) (1)
- Alarm - Home (2)
- Cable TV (2) (3)
- Cell Phone (2)
- Cellar Waterproofing Company (1)
- Clothes Dryer (1)
- Clothes Washer (1)
- Cook Top (1)
- Dishwasher (1)
- Disposal (1)
- Electrician
- Garage Doors
- Heating (and Air Conditioning) (1)
- Housekeeper/Cleaning Service
- Internet Connection (2)
- Kitchen Appliance Installer
- Paving
- Pest Control (1)
- Phone - Landline
- Plumbing
- Range Hood (1)
- Refrigerator (1)
- Television
- Landscaping
- Lawn Sprinklers
- Microwave (1)
- Ovens - Wall or
  Free Standing (1)
- Shades - Motorized
- Shower Glass Enclosure
- Snow Plowing
- Sound System
- Window Cleaners

Other Professionals to Keep Track of:

- Architect

- Builder

- Cabinet Maker and Installer

- Decorator

- Tile Contractor

What Information Is Needed

Where applicable, consider furnishing the following for each item in your chart:

- Name of service or appliance company

- Telephone number

- Name of person you've dealt with before

- Model number

- Serial number

Explanation of Notes

(1) Do you have extended service contracts or extended warranties? If so, where are they, what do they cover and when do they expire? Beside each appliance or item create a symbol to show that extended service benefits apply.

(2) When you call this service provider, you may be asked for a pin number. What is it or where is it?

(3) When you call your cable provider for TV help, they may ask for the serial number of the box that needs help. Here's a place to show it.

CHAPTER 16

Yearly Maintenance Schedule

I can't keep everything in my head, and I excuse this by rationalizing that I have never had a great memory.

Senior years have not improved it. I try to overcome it, but making lists – and "lists of lists," so I have always written things down. And once I see it, I can then organize what needs to be done.

Thus it was very natural for me to go through my calendar last year and create a chart of when house maintenance items were taken care of. From year to year, I add to it, so my survivors will know, as well.

It's that easy.

This chart, table or list should be a month-by-month schedule that alerts your surviving spouse and certainly your executor/executrix as to what needs to be maintained in your home – and when.

Some examples are:

- Heating and air conditioning preventative maintenance

- Turning on and off your lawn sprinklers

- Cleaning gutters

What other mechanisms/chores need yearly attention?

- A sump pump in the cellar if you have a waterproofing system?

- A trap in the laundry that must be filled with water every six months?

- Professional cleaning of the chimney flue?

- If you live in an area where it snows, do you use snow reflectors? Record on a calendar to put them in the ground before it hardens.

- Do you have a contract for snow plowing and do you have to call to confirm arrangements for the coming season?

- Do you have to remind the pest control folks to check out your house or do they arrive automatically?

- And while not exactly "house maintenance," how about a yearly reminder to sharpen your kitchen knives?

CHAPTER 17

Other House Information

There is far more to running a house than fixing appliances and cleaning the windows, as everyday functioning requires knowledge and experience. And while these responsibilities may currently be done by your partner, what happens to YOU, if the situation is reversed? That's why the Guide you are writing needs input from both of you.

Here are subjects, in alphabetical order, which need to be addressed:

Alarm System

- What is the pass code to leave and enter the house, and who else knows this code? Where is the code written down?

- Describe how the system works. What do some of the more important buttons do? Are the sounds for intrusion and fire different? How does your partner sound an alarm in case of panic?

- Who services this system? Their phone number? And when you call, what is the homeowner's code that the alarm company may ask for to be sure they are talking to the home owner and not an intruder?

Deed and Closing Papers for the House

Where are they? Your surviving spouse and certainly your executor/executrix will need them.

Electrical Circuits

Others should know where this panel board is and how to turn off or reset a circuit breaker. There should be a clear listing of the switches and what area(s) each one controls.

Emergency Shutoffs

Boiler There is usually a switch - away from the boiler - that will shut it down in an emergency. Where is it located and under what conditions would you turn it off?

Water <u>Individual Shutoffs:</u> In your basement (or wherever the water enters your home), there are shutoffs for specific outlets – lawn sprinklers, outside faucets, a bath tub, your washing machine, the boiler, etc. Each home is different, but each shutoff should be clearly tagged and the location clearly noted in your *Guide*.

Water <u>Main Shutoff:</u> While this should have a large bright tag on it, take a trip to the basement (or wherever) and show your loved ones where it is. In addition, be sure to state the location in your *Guide*.

Fire Extinguishers

An obvious must for each house; where are yours located? Is the charge current? Who recharges them?

Firearms and Registration

If you have a single firearm or a collection, where is it located? (Use the locator system described in Chapters 25-27.) If you've locked it, where is the key? Is it necessary to register each piece? When and with whom?

Food, Favorites and Fetching

In your relationship, do you purchase certain items for your spouse or vice versa? Examples could be a favorite pie, or where you have clothes dry-cleaned. Which activity or chore is performed by one partner that the other will need to know about when alone?

(A person commented to me that she doesn't think her husband knows where the toilet tissue is stored in the house! And when I told that story to someone else, she said her father-in-law did all the marketing, and when he went on trips, her mother-in-law subsisted on frozen meals and canned goods.)

Gas Grill

How does it work? Self-igniting? Whom do you call for repairs? Any special instructions for changing the tank or winter care? Your partner may handle this now, but your executor may want to know for the next owner.

Heating and Air Conditioning System

In addition to knowing whom to call for service, are there special instructions for proper operation – such as not setting the air conditioning below a certain temperature so the system doesn't freeze up? How many zones are there in the house and what rooms does each zone cover?

Home Improvements

Your accountant will need to know about improvements made, as they can affect taxes you or your estate pays when the house is sold. Where is this information?

Housekeeper

List her (or his) name, address, phone number(s) and partner's name. Does this person have a key and the house alarm code?

Instruction Booklets or User's Manuals for Your Appliances

Over the years, I am sure you have accumulated a bunch of these - mighty handy when new-fangled machines produce annoying beeps and lights, or won't work at all, months or years later. And sometimes, you just need to know which button(s) to push to avoid a costly repair call. Are these booklets in one place? If so, where? If feasible, you can always go online, but be prepared with the name of the manufacturer and model and serial numbers, asked for in Chapter 15.

Keys to the House

Who has a set? It might be wise for your survivor and/or executor to change the locks on your home – then you know. It can be done quickly with radio-dispatched locksmiths, even if it's a pain to redistribute keys to your loved ones and the housekeeper. (Not that she isn't loved, too.) And where are spare keys kept?

Lawn Sprinklers

Yes, the name of the service provider as well as when to call for startup and shut down must be stated, but are there simple operating instructions you can pass on to avoid a costly service call? For instance, should the battery in the unit be changed once a year so if there is a power failure, a service call to reprogram the system won't be necessary?

Locks
Are there any other locks anywhere? If so, where are the keys and who has copies. If the locks are the combination-type, who knows the combination?

Miscellaneous Information on Your Home
Be sure to include anything that is unique to your house – especially if it's something that most houses do not have. Do you have any of the following:

- Lightning rods?

- Cellar waterproofing?

- Special electrical switches such as for a doorbell in the master bedroom?

- Lifetime warranties – for kitchen cabinets, cellar waterproofing, termite control?

Paint Colors
Often a house needs a touch-up – not a whole new paint job, but matching colors can be tricky. Is there any place you have recorded which colors were used? (This should include the paint manufacturer and color name and/or number.)

Paint Disposal
Most communities have rigorous regulations about paint disposal. If you have ever disposed of paint, pass this information along to your surviving spouse so he or she won't have to go through the hassle you did. If it's written, specify where. And of note: communities often have one or two days per year when toxic substances, including paint, can be brought to a named location for disposal.

Pest and Termite Control
What contracts do you have for bug control? With whom? How much do they cost each year? And when paid?

Rented Equipment

I purchased a home only to find out later that the water heater was rented from the gas company. Yes, it should have been divulged long before we closed on the house, but it certainly wasn't worth the chase. So if anything is rented, be sure to place that information in your *Guide*.

Rented House

Do you rent your house to live in or as an investment? If so, how much do you pay? Is there a lease? Where is it and when does it end? Do you receive a monthly bill or just send a check? Who pays for utilities, trash pickup, and snow removal?

Safe – in House

If you have one, what's in it? And where is the combination and/or key to be able to open it up without calling a professional? Who else knows all this?

Voting

Where do you vote? What are your US, state and city congressional districts and wards?

CHAPTER 18

Dates To Remember

As I've gotten older and more of our friends are single, there is a greater need to reach out, to maintain relationships - so that they can enjoy the company of another person or couple and avoid being alone. One way to stay connected is to remember their special events – some of which your partner may know and others you may be familiar with. Why not pool your information so that your partner won't forget these dates?

Create a list which will include:

- The name and address of the person

- The occasion
  (Birthday, anniversary, holidays - such as Christmas, Easter or Thanksgiving)

- The date the card should arrive

- The year that certain events occurred
  (Births, marriages or anniversaries - so that milestones can be acknowledged in a special way.)

How to create such a list? Here are some sources:

- Calendars that your partner or you have kept on the computer or on paper

- People who have remembered you

- A list from which you've sent holiday cards

- Your memory

- By casually asking relatives and friends

Once the information is entered into the chart, I sort it by date (see Chapter 28 and the appropriate index) so it is in chronological order. And another trick I have learned in my old age: On the 15th of each month, my calendar reminds me to buy cards for the following month. Works like a charm.

CHAPTER 19

Computer Information

If you are like me, you have a zillion passwords for all the websites you visit. And have you ever pushed a key on a computer and then had that sinking feeling that you've just screwed it all up? I've also downloaded stuff I wish I hadn't, and my computer crawls. That's when I call in a "geek" to help, but I know whom to call. You do, too, so tell your loved ones about those passwords and helpers. Just be sure the information is secure, as suggested in Chapter 9.

Passwords for Computers

What good is a computer if you can't use it? Start off this chapter in your *Guide* with the password for each computer, if it is required. And if not, mention that as well.

Passwords for Websites

Some people are smarter than I and have the same password for all sites, but I could never figure out how to do that, because one site insists on "six to eight characters with at least 2 digits" and another one is case sensitive while the first one was not. So I have many passwords, and if you are like me, you have a list somewhere of the passwords to the individual sites.

If these passwords are not helpful to your surviving spouse, maybe they will be to the person she may ask to do the bookkeeping or certainly will be to your executor or executrix, who can save lots of time using the Internet to obtain information about your checking and investment accounts. A table of passwords should include:

- The name of the website

- The user ID – additionally called a screen, user, log- or sign-in name

- The password – may be case sensitive so write it down exactly as it needs to be entered in the computer

Security Questions

Many websites want to be sure it's you, so in addition to the password there may be a security question, and you know the answer. So this chart should show:

- The name of the website

- The question that will be asked. Some examples: name of your college, street you were brought up on, mother's maiden name

- The answer

H E L P !

Do you have experience with people who will come to the house to help solve computer issues? Some cable companies and big box stores provide these services, so list them. Besides, there are a bunch of companies with "Geek" in their names.

- Who have you used in the past and what is the contact information?

- How much does it cost and what is the service based on? By the hour? By the project? Any minimum for a house call?

Contracts for Software

First, state the location of the list that contains the contract information. For each one, your *Guide* should answer the following questions:

- Is the contract for hardware or software?

- What computer(s) or program(s) does it cover? What is the telephone number for service? Is the contract for an unlimited or for a given number of calls?

- What is the annual cost, the date of expiration, and how is the contract renewed? Is a bill sent or is it automatically charged to your checking account or credit card?

- If a computer or program is not presently covered, do you know how to obtain a contract in case your partner wants one?

Backup of Information

If you do this, either on a weekly or monthly basis – or both, where are the backups located? Which files are backed up? How are they labeled so if someone wants information from four years ago, he or she isn't the victim of a game of hide and seek?

CHAPTER 20

Electronics in Your Home

The folks who design TVs, cable systems and recording devices are unquestionably electronic wizards, and maybe your partner is also, or maybe he or she is technologically disadvantaged and doesn't care to learn about it or do it because he or she's got "you." To avoid a repeated, "Honey, will you do this for me?" or total frustration, I have placed into writing step-by-step information on how to use some of the features of our sound, television and recording units. It has reduced stress. Maybe it can for you.

You've already listed repair persons in Chapter 15, but here are reminders related to household electronics for which you may have gathered knowledge, being the person who takes care of technology.

Television Problems

When you call the repair person (and you may want to note them here again), is there a pin number needed for identification? What is the number of the cable box giving you a problem? My own *Guide* includes help on these issues:

- How to correct the mistake of shutting off the cable box instead of the TV.

- What to do when there is no data along the bottom of the screen telling you the channel, name of the program and the time.

- How to restart ("reboot") the cable box.

- How to use Caller ID to show incoming calls on the bottom of your TV screen.

Maybe you can think of others – based upon your experience.

Sound System

If you have a system that receives sound from different sources (CDs, a radio, or your computer) and can play it in different rooms, you will need to describe how this system works overall.

My own *Guide* describes our system, first by identifying where the sound comes from and which knob on which unit changes it, so it states:

If the tuner reads...	Then the sound comes from...
CD	The CD player - middle unit*
FM/AM	FM or AM radio - the bottom unit*
VAUX	TV in master bedroom
DVD/VDP	Computer
VCR	WiFi Radio
* as stacked up in my office	

I've recorded that the small unit on top is a distribution box and determines where the sound will <u>be heard</u>. Each button is marked, but starting from the left, the buttons (which may be used in any multiple) are: my office, living room, master bedroom and master bath.

Recording Devices

To me, there is no meeting of the minds of engineers when it comes to recording devices – as every manufacturer or cable provider has its own system – and never the twain shall meet. This applies to DVD and DVR units; a TV that can play a DVD; as well as cable companies, who, needless to say, have their own way of doing things.

Everyone's configuration is different and you may not be as detail oriented as I am, but perhaps now is a good time to orient your partner and share control of the technology, as it can seem very complicated. What follows is an example from my *Guide* of the step-by-step instructions some may attempt to set down. I have treated each unit separately.

First, I determined which functions we use that had to be described and these included:

- Recording, playing, and erasing programs on the system provided by our cable company, and this included scheduling all future programs or only the next one

- Watching a DVD within a combination TV/DVD unit, how to return to the TV screen and get the DVD out of the machine

- Playing the DVD in a separate unit, how to return to the TV screen and get the DVD out of the machine

Each function requires its own chart, but here's an idea of what I used in my *Guide*, but maybe you'll create an easier one.

To Do What?	Remote To Use	What To Do
To play DVD	(1)	Turn on TV
	(2)	Turn on DVD using green button marked "i/o" in upper right hand corner; the red light on the DVD player will turn from red to green. Two buttons to the left of i/o button, use the "open/close" button, open the tray; insert DVD in tray face up. Close tray.
(1) Name of cable company, which appears on the remote (2) name of TV manufacturer which is on the remote		

Section 2
Part C
Downsizing

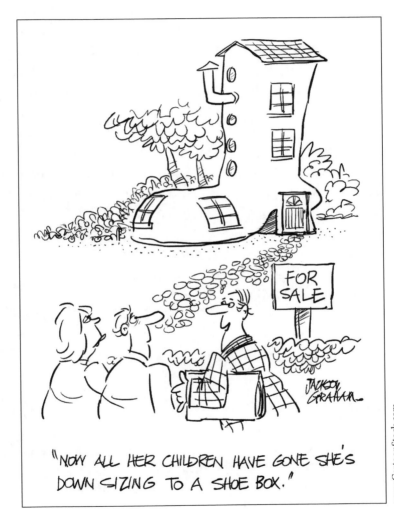

"NOW ALL HER CHILDREN HAVE GONE SHE'S DOWN SIZING TO A SHOE BOX."

CHAPTER 21

Downsizing: Making the Decision

The decision for us to downsize took some thought.

On one hand, we were living fulltime in a beach community 30 minutes from Providence, and while our young grandchildren enjoyed "Camp Rosen," they grew up, and the house became too big. In addition, the drive between our home and our cultural activities in Providence became more difficult in our senior years.

On the other hand, we faced a unique problem as many Rhode Islanders believe that moving to another zip code is moving to a foreign land.

However, we also wanted to be in a home with open-plan living, where the kitchen, dining and living areas are combined (a "great" room) in order to be with each other.

So back to the city we moved.

General Thoughts

Downsizing is certainly a daunting task. What an upheaval! How do you know or will your partner know when it's the right time to downsize? Where to move? How to get rid of the stuff that's been saved? You will need to think about the future life of things that you have. Consider what they mean to you and whether or not they will have the same meaning when you're not around.

Begin to answer all these questions by Googling: "Home Downsizing" and loads of articles will appear. (Using only the word "downsizing" will bring up *corporate* downsizing and *personnel* downsizing), so be sure to include the word "home," and you will find articles on:

- The pluses and minuses of downsizing

- How to start the process of downsizing

- Home buying and selling – the advantages and disadvantages, market timing and whether to buy or sell first

- Making decisions on downsizing: assessing the layout of a new home, identifying where to put what you want to move, and deciding what to keep and what not to

And exactly what do you mean by "downsizing"? A lateral move to a different area? Moving into a smaller house and realizing some equity to put away? Be sure you know your goals, and tell any professional (attorney, accountant or real estate broker) what you want to accomplish.

In addition, there are other things to contemplate:

- Are you willing to go through the process which could take 6 – 12 months?

- Are you prepared to give away some of your possessions? Can you live with less?

- Would a new location give you what you are missing? Would it support the lifestyle you want?

- Don't you want to make the decision now (downsizing and moving – or not) when you have the time and can make the decision together rather than have your children make it for you?

When to Downsize
There is no set answer for everyone. Timing related to the best seller's market (few houses, many buyers) may come into play, but let's explore the advantages and disadvantages.

Advantages of Downsizing

All of these benefits are possible, but may depend upon whether you relocate to a smaller house in a new neighborhood or to an active senior community or assisted living facility.

- Closer to loved ones and friends

- Closer to your medical facilities (or you gain a lot of help with taking and ordering medication if in an assisted living situation)

- Increased cash flow which will provide more money to live on, travel, dine out, etc.

- Fewer rooms and easier to clean, which means more time to do what you want – hobbies, read, etc.

- Minimized stress about money, cleaning and maintenance

- Reduced consumption – less space reduces the urge to buy clothing, groceries and household ornaments

- Less responsibility if you buy a condo

- A home without physical challenges (i.e., stairs, steep walk way, etc.)

- A fresh start, no painful memories within the four walls

- Greater sociability, opportunity to make new friends, join a fun, stimulating senior center

- Being closer to a loved one in a nursing home

- Nearer to your community or cultural activities

- Fewer belongings for the kids to dump because, really, no one wants them

Disadvantages of Downsizing

- Less room for guests – or maybe none at all

- Less space for clothes, groceries and books

- Your new home may not be as prestigious since it's smaller

- You or your children are emotionally attached to your current home

- Need to be more organized

- If a new town, not feeling as safe and secure due to unfamiliarity, not knowing neighbors

- Needing to find new, trustworthy people to help fix or maintain things around the house

- Feeling isolated from friends, not feeling comfortable socializing or taking in lectures, concerts, and other intellectual stimulation because initially you may not know anyone

- New home not conducive to owning a pet, so what will happen to him or her?

And one issue that may be a plus or a minus: You will be leaving one living space (and possibly geographical area) and going to another one. Does this mean a change of lifestyle? And is this a good thing or a bad one or just plain scary?

CHAPTER 22

Downsizing: Further Considerations

Circumstances may impact your decision whether to downsize or not. We had another consideration: Myrna was scheduled for a total knee replacement in the future. So her health and comfort were obviously major deciding forces. But start we did – knee or no knee – because we wanted to move back to the city and it was time to downsize, and we wanted to have the move behind us.

How to Start

You can begin by reading a short, excellent article entitled, "11 Tips to Help You Start Downsizing Your Home," by Michael Ivankovich, which talks about the difficulty of downsizing, and the time and attitude required for the process. Google the title to read it.

Another way to begin the process is to ask a local realtor for some help in organizing. Possibly he or she does it him/herself or can recommend someone whose livelihood is helping others downsize or just get organized. You'll also want to know what your real estate agent thinks your current house is worth. For this reason and for those explained below, a paragraph on "How to Choose a Real Estate Agent" is found in this chapter.

Or, you can start by walking around your home and mentally assessing which rooms you can do without: an extra den, guest room, bathroom, or parlor? Perhaps measure your current living space and decide if you could live with a dining room that is smaller by several feet, a smaller bedroom, etc. This may give you a "rough cut" of what size your new home should be. Remember that you will be giving away or selling clothing, furniture, and everything you've squirreled away in an attic or basement and haven't used for at least a year. Don't forget about paper and canned goods that can be given to a food pantry, as well as dishes, linens and books that you won't need. (For more information on where to donate almost anything, see Appendices B and C.)

How about that stuff you are storing for your kids? Afraid to give them a date to take their belongings off your hands? See Step 4, "Create a Timetable or Schedule," in Chapter 24 to help you. The timetable will give you a reason to prod your loved ones so you can stay on your schedule.

How long do you need to maintain those tax records? Ask your tax professional when you can throw out/shred all that paper. See Appendix A for what to keep and for how long. And do you still cherish those collections that once were so important? Now is the time to scale back.

Downsizing Help

Does this sound intimidating? Do you feel overwhelmed with everything that has to be done? Then get help! Organizations that specialize in this field include:

- Senior Move Managers™, who can help you with an overall plan to downsize - organize and sort out your stuff, assist with measuring furniture and the new floor plan, and just about everything else including unpacking and setting up the new house – or create an "age in place" plan for you.

  The website of their national association is:

  www.nasmm.org

- A search of the Internet produced many "Professional Downsizers," but each one was in a particular area and thus was not appropriate to note here. However, there is a National Association of Professional Organizers and their referral service is:

  www.napo.net/referral

For further sources of help, Google: "senior move managers in *your state*," to bring up websites for other organizations which can help make the job easier.

Downsize to What?

The choices are many, ranging from another private residence to a nursing home (should it be needed). You may even consider moving in with children. But let's look at just two places, if you want to continue being a homeowner and are in good health: a single family home and a condo. Here is a review of the pros and cons of each:

	Advantages	Disadvantages
Home	Total control over your premises	Unexpected major repairs
	Privacy – less noise from neighbors	Higher utility bills due to more space
	Greater choice in layout	More time and expense for upkeep
	Private outdoor space – a place for kids to play outdoors	
	Probably better value – more space for the dollar	
Condo	Lower maintenance bills – especially outdoors – no exterior repairs	Noise of close neighbors
	Someone else takes care of landscaping, snow and ice removal	Decisions made by group for building projects
	Community sociability	Rules and restrictions
	Amenities – could include concierge, gym, pool or sauna	
	If in the city, good views if on a higher floor	
	If a downtown location – closer to restaurants, theaters and concerts	

In addition, there are places with a built-in community and varying levels of care, but there seem to be three basic categories:

- Independent living – provides meals and activities

- Assisted living - provides nursing assistance, in addition

- Nursing home care

If all three types of living are found on one campus, it may be called a Continuing Care Community.

Sometimes these names are bewildering, as the same types of facilities may use different names. To try to make sense out of all this, search the following website:

and then click on (1) "Resources" on the horizontal ribbon, (2) "Articles" on left, and (3) "Types of Senior Living and Care." The article lists the types of personal care offered as well as community services and activities that senior housing can provide.

Explore another explanation of choices at:

www.helpguide.org

Click on "Senior Housing" at the bottom of the left panel, and then on "Understanding Senior Housing Options" in the "Learn About" panel.

This article lists the types of personal care offered as well as community services and activities that senior housing can provide.

For yet a different slant, the website at Seniors For Living™ defines the various types of housing and compares housing types with services provided. You can use this list of possibilities to be sure you end up with what's best for you. Their chart is shown at:

www.seniorsforliving.com

For further sources of help, Google: "senior move managers in *your state*" to bring up websites for other organizations which can provide additional information.

Downsize to Where?

You may have already answered this question, but here are some thoughts:

- Where are your children, grandchildren or friends located?

- Is the weather important?

- Where is the facility - housing community or medical institution that has what you need?

- What are the financial costs of different areas?

There's even a magazine, *"Where to Retire,"* devoted to this subject.

How to Choose a Real Estate Agent

A good real estate agent can be a great source of help in deciding what to do – not only if you should downsize at all – but also in choosing a new type of housing, a different location and other issues that are discussed in this chapter.

In addition, buying or selling your home will be one of the most important financial decisions you make in your life, and a competent real estate agent can make a big difference in outcomes. But before you seek an agent, there are some "designations" you need to know and issues that you must decide for yourself.

Designations of Real Estate "Agents"

On the basic level is a <u>salesperson</u>, who, having passed an exam, has a state-issued license to sell real estate and who works for a broker. Having more experience and professional education is a <u>broker</u>, who can own his or her[6] own real estate company.

A <u>Realtor</u>®, the top professional designation, and required by many agencies, is a member of the National Association of Realtors (NAR) and must abide by their code of ethics. To complicate it further, people who sell real estate are collectively called "agents," as they are in this book.

Questions to Ask Yourself

- <u>Your needs</u>: If you are buying, what's on your wish list? Include medical facilities, house layout, schools, shopping and highway access as well as location, location, location.

- <u>Experience</u>: Do you want a veteran agent or some bright-eyed and bushy-tailed person for whom you are the most important sale of her[6] life? If you are new to the real estate market, a veteran may be better, but an agent with this experience will be juggling many listings, may be more difficult to communicate with, and may have a partner or an assistant with whom you will be dealing. If so, who does what? Yet these experienced veterans probably have a super network of referrals – from their business connections, community activities and social contacts.

6. According to the National Association of REALTORS® report of May 2011, 57% of all REALTORS® are female, and thus future references are "her" rather than "him."

If you choose a newer agent, you might be able to speak to the office manager to determine if the manager is willing to supervise the transaction. (An agent can be considered "newer" if she has been in the business for less than a year or has handled less than two transactions on the buyer's side and two for the seller in the past year.)

- Communication: How much interaction do you need with your agent? If buying, do you want to be called every time a new listing comes on the market? And if selling, every time the house is shown? And how do you want to be contacted? Phone? Email? Texting? Facetime? Just a hand-written note left when the house is shown?

- Seller's vs. Buyer's Agents: Do you care about engaging a seller's or a buyer's agent? Maybe you should. While every agent has a fiduciary responsibility to tell the buyer every thing known about the house – both good and bad, a seller's agent must relate back anything that will help the seller – including what a prospective buyer says, so be careful with your comments.

  And it should be obvious that the agent on the "For Sale" sign in front of a house, the listing agent, is more-over, a seller's agent who will be communicating directly with the seller, and her responsibility, within ethical and legal standards, is to obtain the maximum price for the house.

  When selling, having a competent agent in whom you have confidence is especially important, so the buyer does not come back to you after the sale.

  On the other hand, a buyer's agent has a full responsi-bility to the buyer, and the buyer's agent represents the buyer's best interests including the lowest possible price. So if you are buying, select the agent first so you will know you have someone on your side.

- Chemistry: Does there need to be chemistry between the agent and yourself? Do you think your agent will listen and explain things to you? Will it bother you if this person drives like a nut or constantly says, "like" or "you know" or chews gum while talking?

How to Begin to Choose a Real Estate Agent

- Ask friends who they worked with.

- Ride around the neighborhood and see whom others are using.

- Surf the net - a great tool to evaluate different agencies. If you are buying, how much information is provided in their listings? Schools? Shopping? Highway access? House floor plans? Some agencies allow you to do a "lifestyle search" which allows you to state how important these and other issues like population density or family friendliness are to you. And then the website will suggest communities and properties to you.

Questions to Ask a Prospective Agent

- What experience does the agent have with the neighbor-hood, type of property and price range that you're interested in? How long has she been in the real estate business?

- Is the agent a Realtor®? Has she earned any professional designations, which indicate an advanced level of experience and/or education?

- How many houses (comparable to what you want to buy or sell) were listed or sold by the agent or agency last year? Of those sold, what was the average number of days it was on the market? And what was the percentage of the selling price to the original asking price?

- Why is this agent different from others in the agency? Or from the competition?

- Will the agent work on a timetable that meets your needs (if school schedules or work transfers are an issue)? Does the agent work full time? What hours is she available?

- If you are selling, how will your home be marketed? What tools will be used? Photographs? Video? Staging (see below)? Open house? Floor plans?

- Are there any other services that the agent performs – such as references for house inspections, appraisals or reputable lending professionals or real estate attorneys?

- Can you see a blank copy of the contract the agency wants you to sign? For how long is there exclusive representation? What is the agency's cancellation policy?

- Can you obtain references from people for whom the agent has worked in the past year?

- What is the percentage commission?

Issues in Making Your Choice

- Be sure to read the fine print in the contract before you sign it.

- Don't base your choice solely on a reduced fee. Search around and determine what agents are charging. Remember that a difference in a fee of 1% on a $300,000 sale is $3,000. But won't a good agent/negotiator more than make that up? Unquestionably, $3,000 is more important to your agent than it is to you, as agents are humans, as well, and need to make a living. (Yes, I know, not their entire yearly salary just on your sale.) But don't be afraid to ask your agent to justify her commission.

- Be sure to interview each prospective agent face-to-face before agreeing to representation.

- There's a website that rates (some) agents. Determine if the one you are thinking of choosing is listed:

Lastly, there are two good articles available online. To access the first, search: "How to Choose a Real Estate Agent by Sylvia Booth Hubbard." (It's on the "bankrate.com" website.)

And Google: "How to Choose a REALTOR by the National Association of Realtors®." (This is the "realtor.com" website.)

Purchase or Rent

There is another consideration: do you want to purchase or rent? Again, weigh the pros and cons:

	Advantages	Disadvantages
Rent	Less maintenance responsibility	Could be asked to move at the end of a lease
	Moving out is easier - no responsibilities at end of lease	No rent control unless you have a lease
		No tax benefits
	Landlord pays for costly repairs	
		No build-up of equity
Purchase	Building up equity in your property	Cost of maintenance
	Maintaining the property as you like	Cost of uncontrollable property taxes
	Freedom to change interior and exterior	Less mobility than renting as moving depends on the sale of your house and the purchase of a new one
	Sense of belonging to an area or community	If one has financial problems, loss of house through foreclosure

Buying or Selling Your Home First?

This is an age-old question like the chicken and the egg. You will get as varied an answer as the number of people you speak with. (Maybe you'll get even more answers as some people will say, "Well, if you do this…, but if you do that…" And that's no help at all!) After a while it seems that many of the considerations revolve around time, personal factors, and of course, money – issues discussed here so you can determine your best course of action. You will get heartburn either way, but what's the best for you and your family?

Selling First

Money becomes less of an issue in this scenario because:

- The offer on your house must have been too good to pass up – especially if it's a buyer's market.

118

- You know how much money you can spend on your new home.

- There won't be financing costs - either for a bridge loan or for mortgage payments on the new house (assuming there wasn't a mortgage before).

- You will have the money for a down payment.

- It places you in a stronger bargaining position to buy a new home as financing is not an issue.

- You don't have to maintain two houses.

However, there are disadvantages to selling first:

- You could be homeless. If you have to close on your current home and haven't found a new one, it will be necessary to move into temporary housing.

- In that case, you may have to pay to store your possessions.

- And you may have double moving costs.

- You may not have access to your clothes - if they are stored during a change of season – or be able to get to your papers, if you have the need.

- You could feel pressured to buy something that's not exactly what you want because you've sold your house and have no place to go.

Buying First

On the other hand, there are benefits to buying first:

- You will know the amount of equity you need to get out of your current house to pay for the new one. While that will not influence what someone is willing to pay for your current house, it may help you determine what you're willing to take for it.

- The price on a new house is just too good to pass up.

- You now have a guideline for closing on the current house.

- There may be less pressure to sell your current home as you've financed the new one.

- In a seller's market, houses usually sell more quickly, so you might be willing to gamble that yours will as well.

- Since there's a place to go to, you won't have to move twice.

- You can renovate and move into your new house when it's ready – rather than when you need to – and without living with workmen.

And, again, some negative aspects to consider:

- Are you able and willing to finance two houses?

- Will your bank give you a mortgage if you have one for your current house?

- There will be insurance and maintenance costs to pay on both houses.

- Will you receive low-ball offers on your current house because prospective buyers think you need to sell?

Some Conclusions on Buying vs. Selling First
In deciding which way to go, selling first is probably your option if money is a limiting factor and you have the correct attitude for moving into temporary quarters. Also consider this option if you receive an impressive offer in a buyer's market.

Yet, it seems you should buy first if you can afford to, have the emotional fortitude for carrying two houses, (or have a place to move into temporarily) or if you think your house will sell quickly. In any event, there are things you can be doing regardless of what your choice is. You can begin to gather information to help you make the right decisions for you – starting with whether to downsize or not, buy or rent a new home, and lastly, sell or buy a new home first.

- Call a responsible and active real estate agent and get some professional advice.

- Investigate the possibility of a bridge loan or line of credit if you are willing and able to carry two houses.

- Locate temporary housing. Rent a condo or an apartment?

- Determine what storage will cost. And are there prohibitive policies about when and where possessions can be delivered? How much does it cost to get something out of storage?

Do the math. What's easiest and most convenient for you? Which costs less? For what period of time? Take a guess and double it. Are you still OK with your decision and its costs?

If so, go for it!

Selling Your House

Special Features
If and when you decide to sell your current house, be sure to emphasize why your home is different and its special features. Your real estate agent will work with you to highlight your home's advantages.

Staging
This is a relatively new field in which a professional stager makes your home more appealing after you've cleaned, decluttered, painted, and made minor repairs. To learn more about what staging can do for you, Google: "Home staging Elizabeth Weintraub," or the website of the National Association of Realtors, where there are many articles:

www.realtor.org

Enter, "home staging" in the realtor.org search box for the articles.

There are those who have taken courses in this field, passed exams and are identified when these initials appear:

- ASP® - Accredited Staging Professional
- ASPM® - Accredited Staging Professional Master

To learn more about these designations, you can explore:

www.stagedhomes.com

There is, in addition, an International Association of Home Staging Professionals whose website is:

www.iahsp.com

The Layout of Your New Home

From realtors I know (there are three generations of realtors in our family), there are good layouts and bad ones, so while you're looking, keep this in mind. It could help resale value.

First, a good layout will have:

- **Large Areas for People to Gather:** Family members and friends need space in which to have a conversation.

- **Open Space:** A big, open space gives the impression that the house is larger than it may be.

- **Lots of Natural Light:** People just feel better on sunny days and a house full of natural light gives the same good feeling.

- **Master Bedroom Separate from Other Bedrooms:** Everyone wants privacy for a master bedroom.

And bad layouts include:

- **Inside Stairs Opposite the Entrance:** Not only is it bad feng shui[7] because it allows the energy of the house to escape, but many people are turned off when met immediately by a staircase.

- **Dining Rooms in the Center:** Do you have to walk through this room to get to another one? It's awkward to navigate around the dining room table.

7. An ancient Chinese system to help improve life by receiving positive energy flow.

- **Connecting Bedrooms:** Appraisers consider the two to be one bedroom because of lack of privacy and since each bedroom does not have its own entrance from the rest of the house.

- **Bedrooms Directly off the Living or Dining Room:** There is a noise factor, and again, lack of privacy.

- **Poorly Located Guest Bathrooms:** If far from the guestroom, it could be inconvenient or disorienting for guests at night.

- **Isolated Living Rooms:** This placement can give one a feeling of being disconnected.

Accessible and Universal Design

We are all familiar with the "Handicap Accessible" sign and what it means. Now there's a "universal design" description, which means that the building or product can be used by all.

For instance, a set of stairs to an entrance might have a ramp for the less-abled. That's accessible. But if there were no stairs at all, but rather a level entrance, it would be universal. This can apply not only to entrances, but to family restroom facilities that include a larger space with a changing table or products that make it easier for left-handed people. Other examples include electrical outlets that are higher than normal or using levers instead of round door or faucet handles that require a tight grasp.

CHAPTER 23

Why Organize Your Downsizing and How to Make It Easier

When Myrna and I decided to downsize several years ago, there were many decisions to make.

Among the easiest was finding a new house in the section of the city in which we wanted to live.

The more difficult choices: identifying everything that had to move, establishing a pecking order for giveaways and creating a timetable that met our needs. These are discussed in this chapter and the next.

Once we decided what we were going to use or sell or keep, the decision of who got what became the most challenging. But when we discovered that charities actually wanted what we didn't, it made our decisions easier since so much could be recycled or donated to worthy causes, rather than given to a consignment store, or worse yet, to the junk man. The discovery of this information prompted me to include what I've learned in this chapter, the next, and in the appendices.

Why Organize?

There are many reasons to go through the exercise of identifying the current and future location and size of each piece of furniture – even though it is a pain in the neck. Consider:

- If you are moving a piece of furniture (or rug or lamp, etc.) to your new home with the help of an interior designer, he or she will need to know the size of each piece so that it fits properly.

- Your grandchildren and children will want to know sizes, as this will help them decide if they "need" this piece or not.

- And the same holds for charities.

- Once your grandchildren and children have decided what they want (if anything), you can review the list to be sure you are satisfied with it. Will it cause problems of jealousy later? It's too late once they take it.

- The more you plan, the less time you do without TV or Internet service and the sooner you enjoy a working kitchen – in your new home.

- You will reduce your moving costs by organizing how the mover loads the truck(s) – especially if there are multiple pick ups and/or multiple deliveries. What goes on the truck first comes out last – or sits on the sidewalk for a while!

- By deciding in advance and on paper where everything will go, you are less likely to have something end up in the wrong place – or in the wrong room, and if you are downsizing, you are probably not in a position to do any lifting to correct the mistake.

- Moving can be chaotic. You will be going in a million directions at once, replying to questions that only you know the answers to. The more you plan and tell people in advance and in writing, the less confusion – and stress - on YOU!

How to Make Downsizing Easier

Actions that make the tasks of downsizing manageable:

- Realize that this will take time, and plan on it. Start planning and getting into it long before you think you should.

- Work for only a given period of time per day, then do something else. You may want to tackle this for only one or two hours a day. Just begin.

- Start with a room that you use infrequently – the attic or basement – because it's easier to make decisions with items you don't use every day.

- Keep a side list of items you really want to keep – though the list will become long and you may have to revise it. We have to face that everything won't fit if we are moving into a smaller house.

And as you walk down memory lane, make notes of your family recollections. Your children and grandchildren will thank you.

Once you've made the choice to downsize and have found a place to move into, the ugly question arises of *what do we do with all this stuff?* But this can be done by following 4 easy steps outlined in the next chapter.

CHAPTER 24

Orchestrating That Each Piece Ends Up in the Right Place - in 4 Easy Steps

I simply didn't know how to insure that everything would be moved to the right place. And how to determine there was a fair distribution of furniture among our children and grandchildren?

It finally hit me: do it on paper and in advance, and then I could be sure that everyone was happy. In addition, our decorator gave us a clue when she suggested that we go to the storage warehouse where our furniture was stored and take measurements of each piece.

My ability to make an inventory list on the computer merged those two ideas. And I'm happy to share the process with you.

Considerations in Moving Possessions

- Decide What You Actually Need. This requires being realistic about how you live. Do you truly need 12 place settings of dishes? How about all those books, towels and sheets?

- Measure Your Furniture. For a more detailed explanation, see Step 1 below, identifying everything to be moved.

- Evaluate New Storage Spaces -relative to what you have now. Take a good look in your attic, basement and closets. Don't forget bathroom cabinets and kitchen "junk" drawers and assess which stuff you can do without.

- Dispose of What You Can NOW. Either use it, sell it, give it away, or junk it, but don't move it. Step 3 below - Destinations - will give you more ideas. And don't forget to get your kids to take their stuff – a subject covered in Chapter 22.

- Label Each Box with its destination so it ends up in the right place. It will be easier and quicker to unpack.

- Color Coding. If others are packing for you, place color-coded tags or stickers corresponding to the future destination of each piece so that it, too, is moved correctly. Again, Step 3 delves into this subject in detail.

- Move Large Pieces First - to be sure they are going to fit.

- Unpack Directly. As you unpack a box, place items directly where they are going - into a drawer, cupboard or closet.

And remember to notify everyone of what you're doing by advising them of your new address and telephone number!

Furniture Distribution – An Overview
There are four steps, which make moving, selling, donating and junking easier when downsizing:

1. Identify with a photo and number what is to be moved – regardless of where it is now – and note its dimensions.

2. Create an inventory list showing the current location of each piece and its measurements.

3. Create a prioritized list of the destination of each piece and add this information to the inventory.

4. Make a list of everything to be done which will produce a timetable or schedule.

Step 1: Identify with a Photo WHAT Is to be Moved

Take a photograph of each and every item. In addition to furniture, include tables, lamps, moveable rugs, pieces of art, TVs, computers and printers, anything hanging on the wall, exercise equipment – in short *everything* that has to move, regardless of where it is going, even wall fixtures that are not included in the sale of the house. (If you're not able to take photos, then securely affix numbers to items, room by room, and do a good job describing them in the following chart.)

Prior to taking photos, each item should be arbitrarily assigned a number for identification. Write out the number (large) and put it on the item, so it can be seen in each photograph. My method was to cut an 8 ½ x 11 paper into four pieces, write numbers 0 to 9 boldly on each quarter, and then use them in several photos. For #'s 11, 22, etc., I needed to make some extra numbers.

Next, measure the dimensions of each piece including width, depth and height, as whoever will be using the information (your decorator for your new house, a family member or a charity) will need to know its size. Write the measurements on the back of its photo.

Certain memorabilia deserve separate mention, because they have special meaning. This includes items handed down from parents and grandparents: photo albums, cards, letters, mementoes, or awards or honors from your educational or career experience. Do you have a family history or special collection? Each of these should be photographed and treated as a different item on the inventory (discussed below) to be sure it reaches the desired destination.

Step 2: Create an Inventory Showing Where Each Piece Is Now

It is easy to learn how to create a table on the computer if you take a deep breath and follow the step-by-step instructions provided in Chapter 28 and the appropriate appendix. (And maybe a child, grandchild, or local student can help.) However, feel free to create a binder with this information. You won't have the flexibility to sort different ways, but you'll still stay organized and keep track of your possessions. (If you're doing this on paper, you can skip the location code.) The first step in creating an inventory is to make a list of current locations of everything that has to be moved. It might look like this:

Code	Location Now	Shown in Chart as
1	Cellar	Cellar
2	Living Room	LR
3	Dining Room	DR
4	Kitchen	Kitchen
5	Bedroom #1	Bed #1
6	Bedroom #2	Bed #2
7	Master Bedroom	MBR
8	Den	Den
9	Entry	Entry
10	Outside on the Patio	Patio
11	Mover's Storage Facility	Mover
12	Daughter - Rae	Rae

Why is it necessary to have a location code and a location description? Simply stated, it will reduce errors. If, for example, you were to enter "iving room" for "living room," the entry will not show up with the other "living room" pieces should you sort the list on that column. (Yes, the same is true for a wrong entry of digits, and there it would be even more obvious.)

But don't worry about who gets what. That comes later.

Then create a chart with the headings of the one shown below. For each item for which you have a photo (or will be moving), enter the item number, its description and its three dimensions. The destination codes and destinations will be filled in later.

The inventory list could now look something like this:

Item #	Description	Location Code Now	Location Now	Destination Code	Destination	Width	Depth	Height
1	Table	1	Cellar			48	29	29
2	Lamp	1	Cellar			20	20	28
3	Love Seat	2	LR			52	36	34
4	Couch	2	LR			83	38	30
5	Chest	3	DR			88	20	38
6	Pots/Pans	4	Kitch			x	x	x
7	Bed	5	Bed #1			64	84	28
8	Armoire	5	Bed #1			50	20	65
9	Bed	6	Bed #2			64	84	28
10	Pine Chair	6	Bed #2			24	21	38
11	Bed	7	MBR			80	88	25
12	Mirror	7	MBR			18	18	32
13	Armoire	7	MBR			36	18	81
14	Wing Chair	8	Den			30	33	40
15	Desk Chair	8	Den			20	19	39
16	Red Chair	8	Den			18	17	33
17	Red Table	9	Entry			42	42	30
18	Brass Lamp	9	Entry			16	16	22
19	Wh Furn	10	Patio			x	x	x
20	Grn Furn	10	Patio			x	x	x
21	Table	11	Mover			41	22	29
22	Love Seat	11	Mover			60	33	29
23	TV	11	Mover			80	26	36
24	Wood Chair	12	Rae			26	20	38

You can change this list by sorting on different columns (see chapter 28 and the appendices) so that the order of information – ascending or descending - may be shown by:

- Item number – Have you missed listing a number or an item?

- Current Location – A double check by room that you have accounted for everything.

- Destination – Once this has been established, your inventory tells you who is getting what by sorting on the "destination code" or "destination" column. More on this later.

If you have taken pictures, you will be able to give a set of photos, together with the inventory, to your interior designer or to the prospective recipient so that he or she can decide where to use it or whether to use it at all.

Step 3: Establish a Pecking Order of Destinations

The inventory list will need to show where each item is going. To create a list of destinations, think of what's most important.

First priority – Your Use, Family Use or Later Decision

The top of the list is obvious: What will you be using in the new house? If you engage a decorator, he or she will plan this for you and suggest what can be used although pieces may need to be reupholstered.

There will be pieces you want to keep, but not use right away. I combined those items with those I couldn't make a decision on – yet. And that destination was called "cellar – no decision" – for our later use or consideration; but if you don't have a cellar, have a specific destination in mind - a rented self-storage facility, a moving company warehouse, or the basement of a child.

Once you've decided what you'll use or keep, your grandchildren and children can choose what they want (if anything) by sending them the inventory and a set of photos.

But which family member receives what? Ask each one to give you a list of what he or she wants but ask for a first choice, second choice, etc., in case you have to make a decision. By "giving away" items on paper, you can make changes without causing family problems – possibly giving preference to the grandchildren (over the children) because they are just starting out.

Hopefully, there won't be too many items in contention and each one can receive his or her first choice. By entering destinations determined so far, the inventory will tell you what is not going to be used. That's important as you fill in the chart and complete the process of deciding where everything will go.

Next: What Can You Sell?

This category includes what you can sell to an antiques dealer, at a garage sale, on eBay, on Craigslist, or send to a secondhand consignment shop before or when you move. There are places that will sell your stuff on eBay for you. They will come and get it, sell it on eBay and then keep a percentage of the proceeds. And don't forget to investigate consignment stores for clothes as well as household goods.

A Bit of Caution

Several articles share good advice about selling on either Craigslist or eBay.

- Be sure you know with whom you are dealing. If at all possible, deal with local people.

- Measure and/or weigh the item to determine delivery cost, if that is included in the price.

- List the item as "used" to avoid problems related to the condition of what's being sold.

- Make the terms of sale VERY clear. Does the price include delivery? What is the return policy? What are terms of payment?

- Be sure to obtain a delivery confirmation.

- Don't give out any financial information – including bank account or Social Security numbers.

- If the buyer sends more money than required, be wary of a scheme.

- Don't be the first to give feedback or rate the buyer, because if the buyer berates you afterward, your feedback makes you look bad.

- Use common sense. If in doubt, back out.

If you want to sell books, search for buyers at:

www.bookscouter.com

Bookscouter allows you to search at over thirty-five different book-selling websites, lists potential buyers and the price being offered for your book. Since each book must be entered individually, the site might be used only for your more expensive books.

Recalls

Before you sell or donate something, be sure the item hasn't been recalled, which can be checked at:

www.recalls.gov

Confirm that the item is safe.

What's Your Stuff Worth?

Here are suggestions to help you obtain a realistic value on what you own.

Go onto the eBay website and review completed sales. Other sources to establish current values:

- Craigslist - find out what people are asking

- Browse through antique stores

- Ask auctioneers

- Visit consignment and pawn shops

In addition, Michael Ivankovich has another article in which he talks about ways to determine what your possessions are worth. Read it at:

www.homedownsizingconsultants.com/blog.html

But be sure to obtain values from sources that are independent from anyone connected to the sale. Don't make the mistake of allowing a person to sell your articles just because he or she gave you a high estimate of value. It may have been done to obtain the representation.

Appraisers

There are national organizations which might be able to help you determine the value of your possessions and your home.

- The Appraisers Association of America:

www.appraisersassoc.org

In the upper left, click on "FIND AN APPRAISER." You can then either do a quick search for an appraiser or do a "Specialization Search" for different articles by clicking on "Start Search" next to the appropriate item.

- The Appraisers Society of America:

www.appraisers.org

Click on "Find an Appraiser" on the left.

For a real estate appraiser in your area, Google: "Real estate appraiser in *your city, state,* etc." Some appraisers are certified by the Certified Appraiser Guild, which means they adhere to the Certified Appraiser's Code of Professional Ethics and to the Uniform Standards of Professional Appraisal Practice. More about this designation can be found at:

www.caga.synthasite.com

OK, hopefully you have gotten over the shock of how little your possessions are worth, and the next mental roadblock is to get rid of the balance.

Giveaways

Here, as well, is a pecking order: recycling centers, donations and finally the junk man. Some cities have special dates for curb pick up – including furniture, but before you decide to dump something (which may cost money to cart away), consider that there are many places to recycle and donate stuff, which may result not only in a charitable donation, but possibly more important, in helping someone else.

And since there is so much information on recycling and donations, the subject is discussed generally in this chapter, but Appendix B will direct you to organizations that accept many items and Appendix C lists where to donate specific items. For the moment, either:

- Create a general destination called "giveaways" which means you can review it later when you can be more specific, or

- Become familiar with the organizations now so that when you decide on destinations, you can pop this information into your inventory table.

Recycling

There are several good articles online on recycling:

Article Title	Website
How To Recycle Practically Anything[8]	www.emagazine.com
Recycling More Obscure Materials	www.obviously.com/recycle/guides/hard.html
Things You Might Not Know You Can Recycle[9]	www.thegoodhuman.com

Sometimes when you donate something, the recipient organization may recycle your donated article(s) so you'll be helping the environment, as well as giving a boost to the organization.

In surfing the net, I came across a great website which helps you through this maze:

www.earth911.com

All you do is enter the item to be recycled and your location; the website directs you to the closest place to take your stuff. And "stuff" here means paper, metal, hazardous waste material, plastic, glass, automotive, household, garden composting or construction materials. Also included are electronics – cell phones, computers, empty ink cartridges and televisions.

If you want to recycle *and* sell items, check out:

www.gazelle.com

This organization purchases all kinds of devices including: camcorders, cell phones, digital cameras, GPS devices, iPads, iPhones, laptops, MP3 players, PDAs, satellite radios, video games and XBoxes.

Donating

Before deciding which charities to give your donations to, you should know that a charity is reputable. Use these resources:

- The Better Business Bureau:

www.bbb.org/us/Charity-Reviews

Will aid you in determining if the charity spends its donations as it says it will, if it has good governance practices, or spends too much money on its own expenses.

8. On the eMagazine website, type in the name of the article in their search box, and click on the icon within the box – to the left of the word "login."
9. On the Good Human website, click on Archives, enter the article title in the search box, and click on "search" to read the article.

- Charity Navigator:

www.charitynavigator.org

Evaluates financial health of organizations

- Give Well:

www.givewell.org

Focuses, according to their website, on "how well programs actually work – i.e., their effects on the people they serve."

Many organizations have local drop off points; others have guide lines as to what they will and will not accept. Check out individual websites in Appendices B and C.

To be sure you get a tax deduction, consult a professional, but also Google: "Don't Dump It, Donate It!" at the *Ladies Homes Journal* website to review the tips at the end of the article.

There are specific guidelines to obtain a non-cash deduction, so consult with a tax professional or at least read the article, "How to Value Non-Cash Deductions," on:

www.ehow.com

For furniture, Google: "Furniture Tips Help Needy Families," found on:

www.charityguide.com

Car donations have their own guidelines, so search for "How to Donate Your Car," on:

www.ehow.com

Cell phones are a wonderful donation that can help an abused person or a serviceman or woman. But before you just throw your phone in a "recycle bin" somewhere, there are precautions to take.

- Be sure your phone service is discontinued on the phone(s) you are recycling.

- Erase your personal information; this will be done correctly if a technician at your phone store does it. The "SIM card," (if your phone uses one), will be removed, which is the "guts" or hard drive of the phone and contains your phone numbers, text messages, etc.

- Do you know the charity that is going to recycle it? If not, it may be just scrapped.

Also of note is an organization called The Giving Effect, which identifies charities in your area whose causes you may want to support, and what they accept. This website allows you to choose a delivery preference (mail, their pickup or your drop-off), a cause category (education, health, the military, etc.) and some 33 categories of items to donate:

www.thegivingeffect.com

Click on the "Explore and Donate" tab.

There are other local choices as well: Blankets and heavy towels can be donated to animal shelters, which use them in cages. Ask what your libraries, schools, religious organizations, and family members need.

Here are three articles that I found helpful:

- "Stuff Ya' Don't Want," at

www.stuffyadontwant.com

Click on the item to be given away to locate donation centers for afgans and veggie oil and 50 items in between.

- "Where to Donate All Your Unwanted Stuff," is found by entering the title in the Google search box. The article is on the www.thegoodhuman.com website – for art supplies to magazines to packing peanuts to wire hangers.

- "Don't Dump It, Donate It!" – noted above – should also be Googled. It is found on the website of the *Ladies Home Journal* and is yet another place to donate everything from blankets to sports equipment.

Click on the "Explore and Donate" tab.

Deciding: Who Gets What?

By this point you know the different people or places that will receive your possessions, and you can update your inventory list and assign a code to each destination, doing so in any order that comes to mind. Each room in the new house should receive a different code as should each person – by name. Don't worry about who gets what. That comes next. Here's what our list, abbreviated, looked like just to give you an idea:

Destination Code	Destination	Shown in Chart as
1	New House - Master Bedroom	MBR
2	New House - Guest Bedroom	Guest
3	New House - Kitchen	Kitchen
4	New House - Liv Rm/Dining Rm	LDR
5	No Decision: New House Basement	Base ND
6	Sell before moving - Craigslist	Craigslist
7	Daughter - Sue	Sue
8	Daughter - Liz	Liz
9	Grandchild - Jake	Jake
10	Son - Ben	Ben
11	Secondhand Consignment Store	2nd Hand
12	Upholsterer	Uphol
13	Charity A - by mover	CharityA
14	Charity B - by owner	CharityB
15	Junk Dealer	Junk
16	No Decision - Self Storage	Slf Store
17	Sell before moving - Garage Sale	Gar Sale
18	New House - Office	Office
19	Sell before moving - Antiques Dealer	Antiques
20	New House - Deck/Patio	Deck
21	Recycling Center - Johnston	Recycle
22	Daughter - Rae	Rae

Now for the final decisions.

You've probably already entered the destinations for items going into your new home, being given to your family (having worked with the lists from the kids), and you know which items can be sold or given away. To complete the inventory list, look at which items still need to be matched up with a destination, using notes from any websites you've researched.

Don't worry if you make a mistake. It's just on paper! Make the decision and think about it. Go back and change it. You are making progress!

By filling in the "Destination Code" and "Destination" columns for each item, the inventory will look like this:

Item #	Description	Location Code Now	Location Now	Destination Code	Destination	Width	Depth	Height
1	Table	1	Cellar	5	Base ND	48	29	29
2	Lamp	1	Cellar	14	CharityB	20	20	28
3	Love Seat	2	LR	3	Kitchen	52	36	34
4	Couch	2	LR	22	Rae	83	38	30
5	Chest	3	DR	17	Gar Sale	88	20	38
6	Pots/Pans	4	Kitch	3	Kitchen	x	x	x
7	Bed	5	Bed #1	9	Jake	64	84	28
8	Armoire	5	Bed #1	19	Antiques	50	20	65
9	Bed	6	Bed #2	10	Ben	64	84	28
10	Pine Chair	6	Bed #2	18	Office	24	21	38
11	Bed	7	MBR	1	MBR	80	88	25
12	Mirror	7	MBR	16	Slf Store	18	18	32
13	Armoire	7	MBR	19	Antiques	36	18	81
14	Wing Chair	8	Den	12	Uphol	30	33	40
15	Desk Chair	8	Den	13	CharityA	20	19	39
16	Red Chair	8	Den	2	Guest	18	17	33
17	Red Table	9	Entry	6	Craigslist	42	42	30
18	Brass Lamp	9	Entry	11	2nd Hand	16	16	22
19	Wh Furn	10	Patio	15	Junk	x	x	x
20	Grn Furn	10	Patio	20	Deck	x	x	x
21	Table	11	Mover	4	LDR	41	22	29
22	Love Seat	11	Mover	8	Liz	60	33	29
23	TV	11	Mover	21	Recycle	80	26	36
24	Wood Chair	12	Rae	13	CharityA	26	20	38

If you sort the table on "Destination Code" (column 5), the above list will change to read:

Item #	Description	Location Code Now	Location Now	Destination Code	Destination	Width	Depth	Height
11	Bed	7	MBR	1	MBR	80	88	25
16	Red Chair	8	Den	2	Guest	18	17	33
3	Love Seat	2	LR	3	Kitchen	52	36	34
6	Pots/Pans	4	Kitch	3	Kitchen	x	x	x
21	Table	11	Mover	4	LDR	41	22	29
1	Table	1	Cellar	5	Base ND	48	29	29
17	Red Table	9	Entry	6	Craigslist	42	42	30
22	Love Seat	11	Mover	8	Liz	60	33	29
7	Bed	5	Bed #1	9	Jake	64	84	28
9	Bed	6	Bed #2	10	Ben	64	84	28
18	Brass Lamp	9	Entry	11	2nd Hand	16	16	22
14	Wing Chair	8	Den	12	Uphol	30	33	40
15	Desk Chair	8	Den	13	CharityA	20	19	39
24	Wood Chair	12	Rae	13	CharityA	26	20	38
2	Lamp	1	Cellar	14	CharityB	20	20	28
19	Wh Furn	10	Patio	15	Junk	x	x	x
12	Mirror	7	MBR	16	Slf Store	18	18	32
5	Chest	3	DR	17	Gar Sale	88	20	38
10	Pine Chair	6	Bed #2	18	Office	24	21	38
8	Armoire	5	Bed #1	19	Antiques	50	20	65
13	Armoire	7	MBR	19	Antiques	36	18	81
20	Grn Furn	10	Patio	20	Deck	x	x	x
23	TV	11	Mover	21	Recycle	80	26	36
4	Couch	2	LR	22	Rae	83	38	30

There was now a list by destination of every item, and after sharing with the decorator, it showed that:

- The love seat (item #3) had been misdirected into the kitchen (destination #3). Oh, really?

Other important information we picked up from sorting by destination was that Sue, our daughter, was not receiving anything – no destination #7. Was that her wish, a mistake, or a problem?

- There was only one item for self storage (destination #16), and that wasn't worth it, so the pine mirror would either be moved to the cellar (#5) or added to the garage sale (#17).

Yes, the time allocated to planning and organizing had been well spent.

And while I was at it, I measured the following areas to be sure everything would fit.

- The linear feet required in the kitchen for dishes, groceries and paper goods.

- And the same information for clothing – not only in the bedroom closets, but in the front hall for guests and the back hall for everyday jackets.

- The footage needed for books, linens, and miscellaneous accessories like large serving dishes and even flower pots.

Now, how to get everything in the right place, on time? That's Step 4.

Step 4: Create a Timetable or Schedule
In business, a mark of a good executive is accomplishing a goal within budget and on *time*, and a timetable or schedule has given me the tools to meet these goals. But how to begin?

Just write down on paper, *in any order*, what has to be done and how much time you estimate is needed. Don't really know? Take a guess. *Start backwards!* Establish your finish date first! In the beginning, our list was in no order whatsoever and looked like this:

What Has To Be Done	Time Needed	When To Start	Finish Date
FINISH DATE - unpacking in new house	3 weeks	Dec 10	Dec 31
Send inventory to kids	4 weeks	Before other pickups	
MOVERS PACKING – overnight in hotel	1 day	Day before moving	
MOVING DAY– 1st night in new house	1 day	MOVING DAY	
Personally move fragile items and financial records	3 days	Before move	
New connections: phone, TV, internet and sound at new house	2 days	Before move	
Kids pickup	3 days	Before garage sale	
Junk dealer pickup - pool and garden furniture	1 day	Before the 1st snow fall	
Charities to pick up at old house	4 days	Before move	
Disconnect TV, phone and internet at old house	1 days	Before move	
Clean new house	3 days	After move	
Clean old house	2 days	After move	
Furniture sent to be reupholstered	8 weeks	Before move	
Carpet installed in new house	5 days	Before move	
All contractors OUT of new house (1)	2 days	Before move	
Garage sale	1 day	After kids' pickups	
Antiques dealer picks up – old house	2 days	Before move	
(1) I held on to this date tenaciously, but I knew there was play.			

In our case, I was starting an interim job on the second day of the new year, so December 31st became our finish date. My wife was still recovering from surgery, and I wanted to be sure that I had enough time to unpack all the boxes before then, so I gave myself three weeks to get it done, as you can see in the chart above.

Since the finish date was December 31st and three weeks were needed to unpack in our new home, the move had to be around December 10th. That meant the movers would start to pack on the 8th (2 days for packing and moving according to their estimator) and that determined that I had to move stuff personally on the 7th. My schedule was starting to fill in, and some dates were assigned arbitrarily to find problems.

Our list then showed:

What Has To Be Done	Time Needed	When To Start	Finish Date
FINISH DATE - unpacking in new house	3 weeks	Dec 10	Dec 31
Send inventory to kids	4 weeks	Before other pickups	Sept 15
MOVERS PACKING - overnight in hotel	1 day	Day before moving	Dec 8
MOVING DAY- 1st night in new house	1 day	MOVING DAY	Dec 9
Personally move fragile items and financial records	3 days	Before move	Dec 6
New connections: phone, TV, internet and sound at new house	2 days	Before move	Dec 7
Kids pickup	3 days	Before garage sale	Nov 21
Junk dealer pick up - pool and garden furniture	1 day	Before the 1st snow fall	Oct 15
Charities to pick up at old house	4 days	Before move	Dec 5
Disconnect TV, phone and internet at old house	1 day	Before move	Dec 8
Clean new house	3 days	Before move	Dec 6
Clean old house	2 days	After move	Dec 11
Furniture sent to be reupholstered	8 weeks	Before move	Oct 8
Carpet installed in new house	5 days	Before move	Dec 4
All contractors OUT of new house (1)	2 weeks	Before move	Nov 24
Garage sale	1 day	After kids' pickups	Nov 25
Antiques dealer picks up - old house	2 days	Before move	Dec 7
(1) I held on to this date tenaciously, but I knew there was play.			

Having used a Word® table to create the list, I could then easily sort it by "Finish Date" (the 4th column) which allowed me to place all the activity in chronological order – in short, a schedule! And the problems came into focus:

What Has To Be Done	Time Needed	When To Start	Finish Date
Send inventory to kids	4 weeks	Before other pickups	Sept 15
Furniture sent to be reupholstered	8 weeks	Before move	Oct 8
Junk dealer pick up - pool and garden furniture	1 day	Before the 1st snow fall	Oct 15
Kids pickup	3 days	Before garage sale	Nov.21
All contractors OUT of new house (1)	2 weeks	Before move	Nov 24
Garage sale	1 day	After kids pickup	Nov 25
Carpet installed in new house	5 days	Before move	Dec 4
Charities to pick up at old house	4 days	Before move	Dec 5
Personally move fragile items and financial records	3 days	Before move	Dec 6
Clean new house	3 days	Before move	Dec 6
New connections: phone, TV, internet and sound at new house	2 days	Before move	Dec 7
Antiques dealer pick up – old house	2 days	Before move	Dec 7
MOVERS PACKING – overnight in hotel	1 day	Day before moving	Dec 8
Disconnect TV, phone and internet at old house	1 day	Before move	Dec 8
MOVING DAY– 1st night in new house	1 day	MOVING DAY	Dec 9
Clean old house	2 days	After move	Dec 11
FINISH DATE - unpacking in new house	3 weeks	Dec 10	Dec 31
(1) I held on to this date tenaciously, but I knew there was play.			

Do not use a range of dates, such as "Dec 7-9," as Word® will not recognize it, and the column will not sort properly.

And the schedule told me:

- Action was needed in September (!) for a December move in case any of the kids wanted the pool and garden furniture – to give them time to make decisions and for pickups. But this would be for the outdoor stuff only since it wasn't acceptable to live for two or three months without major pieces of furniture.

- We needed more time between the kids' pickups (November 21st) and the garage sale (November 25th) as possibly someone would want something but needed some time to decide.

- There was obviously too much to do on December 6th, 7th and 8th, so all that had to be spread out. Dates were changed, and the chart sorted again to determine if the actions could be accomplished as shown. This was done as many times as necessary to have a reasonable plan.

I couldn't have gotten all these details straight without a schedule.

You are now ready to get moving – your furniture and yourself. Good luck in your new digs! You've done a mighty good job!

SECTION 3

Helpful Skills For Writing *Your* Own *Guide*

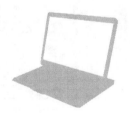

Section 3
Part A
Locating Documents

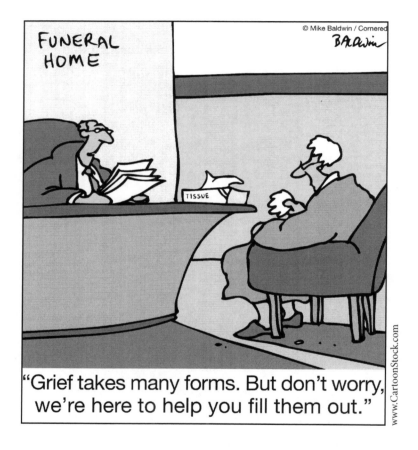

"Grief takes many forms. But don't worry, we're here to help you fill them out."

CHAPTER 25

How to Identify Locations of Documents

As my wife and I age, we find ourselves saying, "It takes two." Two of us to do the things that one of us could do just a few years ago. Yes, she points out stop signs; I prompt her to take her medications; and we help each other recall the first or last name of someone we both know but cannot remember.

Well, your Guide that you write for your partner will be the new "Number Two" – when you're not here.

So for now, the "concept of two" works well since we are both here and my part is knowing where all of our papers and documents are located. But, how can I tell her where to find them when I'm not here? And how to convey this to our executrix who knows even less? To solve that problem, I have developed a simple locator system that you can use to relate where everything is.

I hope you find it helpful and efficient.

Locating documents is <u>not</u> supposed to be a game of hide and seek – where you hide vital information and your loved ones, executor or professionals seek. That becomes costly, both emotionally and financially, so this and the next two chapters will provide tools to help cut down on the time it takes to locate your documents.

While there are many places in a home or office where information can be kept or filed, let's talk first about some of the common areas, and how to describe them, so someone else can find a document quickly.

File Cabinets and Their Drawers

An obvious place to store paper - in drawers and file cabinets - can also prove to be a time waster unless the location is described fully and accurately.

Here's how it can be done easily:

First, state the <u>general</u> location of all the file cabinets or shelves. Examples are:

- under my desk in my office

- in the spare room, on the left as you enter

- in the cellar, to the right of my desk as if you were sitting at the desk

Second, determine the specific place that you are referring to. If there are nine (or less) choices it will suffice to identify them by top-right, top-center, top-left, center-right, etc. However, if you have numerous choices, you may need to be more specific. Let's assume that there are 3 file cabinets – each with 4 vertical drawers. Start by "naming" the cabinets. You could say, "From left to right, I have given each cabinet a letter. The cabinet on the left is 'A', and the one on the right is 'C'. And in each file cabinet, there are four vertical file drawers, and I have numbered the drawers starting at the top and going down as '1', '2', '3' and '4.'" Thus the drawer locations, as you look at them, would be:

A1	B1	C1
A2	B2	C2
A3	B3	C3
A4	B4	C4

Now you can refer to a specific drawer in the same way a spreadsheet refers to a specific cell. And YOU have a simple locator system!

Bookshelves

As said before, relate where the bookshelves are (office, cellar, living room, etc.) and then the bookshelf itself. And assuming you have more than one set of bookshelves, describe exactly where each one is.

For example: "As you walk into my office, there are bookshelves on the center wall above my desk and on the right wall."

Or you could say, "In my office there are 3 vertical bookcase sections over the center part of the desk and 2 vertical sections on the right as you walk in.

Desks

Again, this is a favorite place for documents, but those who will need to find important papers without your help ought to know where to look. So describe and identify the drawers in the same fashion as you did for file cabinets and bookshelves.

The Cellar and Attic

This is a wonderful place to get stuff "out of sight," but it will be costly for those you leave behind to comb through all the records looking for what is needed.

A solution? Buy file transfer boxes at an office supply store, number the boxes, and then inventory what's in each box in a chart in Windows Word®.

Woops! Don't know how to create a chart (or table)? Chapter 28 and the appropriate appendix will tell you how.

But first, it's necessary to give your loved ones an overview of where *your documents* are located. That is the subject of Chapter 26.

Generally, What's Where?

I admit it: When it comes to records and documents, I save them. So much so, I have boxes and boxes of files in my basement. And then there are documents on bookshelves and in file cabinets. Yes, I should go through them and throw half of the stuff out. But I don't – and haven't. To maintain my own sanity in order to find papers quickly, I use an overview suggested here or the list as described in Chapter 27.

A Bird's Eye View

There should be a chapter in your *Guide* describing, generally, what is in each location for which you have developed a locator system – a bird's eye view of that drawer, shelf, file drawer or box. It is also a good place to explain, in brief terms, the contents of various notebooks, if you use them.

For example, you could say, "On the left side of my desk, drawer A1 contains unpaid bills, blank checks, bank checking account statements and other <u>active</u> financial records. Drawer A2 has last year's bills and other records needed for preparing this year's taxes, and drawer A3 has travel stuff – future trips, restaurant reviews and restaurants we want to visit.

"And on top of my desk is a standup file organizer which holds the files I use most often: files on our prescription information, the fundraising effort for XYZ school I'm working on, etc."

Or, "On shelf D2 there's a notebook labeled, 'Misc. Information.' This notebook contains family dates of birth, dates of graduation, magazine subscription expiration dates, and on shelf D3 is the notebook with all our appliance service contracts and whom to call when something doesn't work."

This can be done in as much detail as you want – or as much as you are willing to do to help your loved ones locate papers.

CHAPTER 27

Locations of Specific Documents

So now my survivors know how I've identified the locations and I've given them an overview of what's where. Create your own references similar to the examples shown below, and imagine your survivors' relief to know your affairs were truly put "in order."

Important Documents – The Master List!

Here is a comprehensive list of important documents. Though lengthy, you will be saving a ton of time for your survivors and executor.

Document	Location	Specific Location
Adoption papers	Office shelves	Shelf E2 (1)
Appointment calendar		
ATM cards		
Bills – paid	Cellar	Box 24 (1)
Bills – unpaid		
Biographical information		
Birth certificates		
Burial plot deed		
Business insurance information		
Car leases		
Cell phone leases		
Citizenship		
Civil unions		
Computer information – passwords and contracts		
Court documents for almost anything		
Credit card photostats		
Credit cards		
Divorce decree(s)		
Drivers' licenses		
Drug insurance (Plan D)		
Employment records and benefits		

Document	Location	Specific Location
Eyeglass prescriptions		
Family birthdays, anniversaries and graduation dates		
Final letter(s) to loved ones		
Funeral		
Guardianship(s)		
Heath insurance information		
House purchase(s) and sale(s) (2)		
Index to cellar boxes containing files (3)		
Insurance files		
Investment account reports		
IRAs		
Life insurance		
Magazine subscription expiration dates		
Marriage certificate(s)		
Military service records, number and discharge		
Passport photostats		
Passports		
Power of Attorney – health		
Power of Attorney – use of health information		
Powers of Attorney – legal		
Pre- or Post-nuptial agreements		
Religious records		
Resumes		
Safe – at bank – contents		
Safe – in house – contents		
Social Security numbers – kids		
Social Security numbers – ours		
Tax returns – federal and state		
Trusts		
Wills		
(1) Creating a locator system was described in Chapter 25.		
(2) Former house(s), too.		
(3) This could be a chart or table that lists all individual files in transfer boxes in the cellar		

Section 3
Part B
Creating and Using a Table

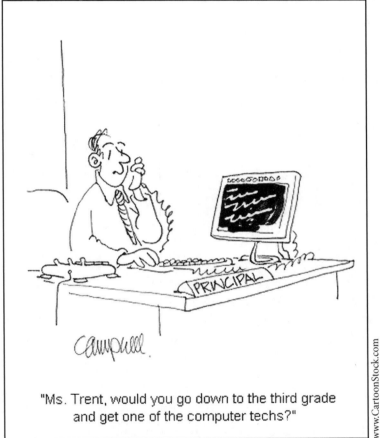

"Ms. Trent, would you go down to the third grade and get one of the computer techs?"

www.CartoonStock.com

CHAPTER 28

Using a Table in Word®

Using Microsoft's Word® to create a document on the computer opened a whole new world to me, as I found it easier to write letters and create lists using this program. But not everyone is comfortable using a computer, and many of my generation have a limited ability to use Word®. This chapter will get you started and depending upon which computer and version of Word® you have, lead you to the appropriate appendix, which will teach you how to create a table as well as other functions that have allowed me to get a lot accomplished quickly.

I am sure it will for you, too.

You may be technologically challenged and find you just don't get along with computers, <u>but don't skip this chapter</u> and the appropriate appendix! Rather, read and try it, and even engage a child, grandchild or local high school or college student to help you understand it. Cutting edge research tells us that to keep our brains healthy and functioning, we need to learn new skills – perhaps think of this as a fun puzzle to solve!

There are many avenues of assistance: you can access a tutorial within your computer; attend a course often offered at libraries or local colleges; use Google to learn; inquire in the store where the computer was purchased; or ask your local computer tech or where your computer is repaired. And bookstores offer self-help guides to get you computer literate. If all this fails, <u>then</u> your "teacher" can guide you or do the work on the computer for you. But it may be easier than you think!

Why Use a Table?

It's much <u>faster to find information</u> in a table than in text, as it is difficult and tedious to pick information out of a paragraph. However, pre-made tables alone do not allow you to add explanatory notes (and your household information is unique), so it's necessary to learn <u>how to create your own table</u>. In addition, a blank space in a pre-made form leaves room for questions.

A TABLE, in Microsoft Word®, is an outline – similar to the old graph paper (am I showing my age?), which shows a variable number of vertical columns and horizontal rows of your choosing, according to your needs. In each "box," called a CELL, you can type words or digits or information of any nature.

Header Row		
1		
1	2	
1, 3	3	3

Graphically,

The "1's" represent a column; the "2" shows a cell, and the "3's," a row.

Using Word® on the Computer

If there is not a "Blue W" along the side or bottom of the "Home" page, get some help. Word® may not be visible to you, or loaded on your computer.

However, if you have opened Word® and don't know which version you have (is anything simple?), use the following commands:

For Macs:
　　2004: Click on **HELP** > **ABOUT WORD*** > **OK**
　　2008: Click on **HELP** > **ABOUT WORD*** > **OK**
　　2011: Click on **HELP** > **WELCOME TO WORD*** >
　　　　　CONTINUE
For PCs:
　　2003: Click on **HELP** > **ABOUT MICROSOFT WORD*** > **OK**
　　2007: Click on **Microsoft Office button** in the upper left part of the
　　　　　screen > **WORD OPTIONS******>RESOURCES** > **ABOUT***
　　　　　> **OK**
　　2010: Click on **FILE** > **HELP*** > Close drop down box.

* The version is shown in this screen.
** WORD OPTIONS is displayed at bottom edge of drop down box.
Here's where the different versions are located in this book:

If you have a Mac:
　　For Word® 2004: Appendix 1
　　For Word® 2008: Appendix 2
　　For Word® 2011   Appendix 3

If you have a PC:
　　For Word® 2003: Appendix 4
　　For Word® 2007: Appendix 5
　　For Word® 2010: Appendix 6

How to Highlight an Area

Many of the functions in Word® require selecting and thus defining
an area. To "highlight" information, place the cursor and click down
before the first letter of the first word, and holding down the mouse,
slide it until the end of the area you want is reached. The area will
appear shaded, possibly in a light color or even blackened.

Or, if your hand, like mine, is not as steady as it once was, place the
cursor and click on the first letter of the first word or digit. Hold down
the **SHIFT** key while using the right arrow key to highlight the area.

To remove highlighting, click on another area.

The use of the word "text" in the appendices includes letters, digits, tables, or whatever.

<u>Explanation of Instructions</u>
When you read, "**EDIT > COPY**," it is shorthand for click on **EDIT** and then click on **COPY** - commands at the top of the screen.

You've gotten this far: Don't give up now. Go to the appropriate appendix and surprise yourself! Then you can brag to the younger generation, "Look what I've learned!"

SECTION 4

Conclusion

BONUS: Download the FREE companion app at www.MyFamilyRecordBook.com

CHAPTER 29

You've Done It!

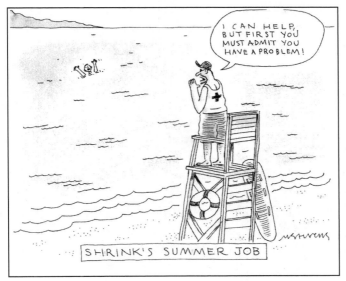

© Mick Stevens New Yorker Magazine/Conde Nast

Congratulations! You've made it through this book, whose purpose has been to prompt a family's current financial and house "manager" to commit to writing all the things in his or her head that a survivor and executor need to know. You now understand how much information you have and how useful it will be to your partner, loved ones, estate attorney and executor(s).

It has been fun writing this book, and it has kept me off the streets.

But it will have served its objective if it has challenged you to think about the future, and changed your frame of mind about the inevitable. The inevitable need not only mean death, but any unfortunate health circumstances that remove your ability to manage your household responsibilities – short term or long.

Are you surprised at how many home and financial responsibilities there are? Possibly the book covers more subjects than you realized warrant attention, but you and I both know it doesn't include everything. So think about what you own, consider the lifestyle you want your survivor to enjoy, and realize that you have made it easier for those who will remain behind.

Yes, congratulations!

You've been there every step of the way – supporting, helping, loving and doing. The *Guide* you will write expresses that you still care, that in a way, you'll still be there, helping and loving them. I particularly hope this book has deepened your concern about the future life of your partner.

It should be obvious that the more information you furnish your professionals (attorneys and accountants), the lower the charges to your estate. As stated in the introduction to this book, why pay a professional to search for information that you have in your head? It's really a slam dunk.

Okay, you've completed the first part of planning how to safeguard the lifestyle of your partner – reading this book. Now finish the task and get all that information in a computer or on paper! And in your words. Your *Guide* will assure you that you have done everything in your power to help your survivors ease into the next stage of life.

The *Guide* you write will give your survivors and executor as much confidence to face the future as you are able to provide, and that has to make you feel good. But before you pat yourself too hard on the back, stop reading and start writing. Then you can truly pat yourself on the back. And you will! I know I have, and the feeling is really, really good.

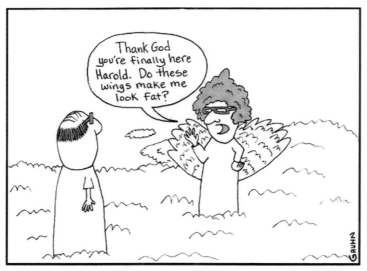

Appendix A
What to Shred and When

Never:
- Social Security card
- Papers for the purchase, improvements, or sale of homes, vehicles, or boats
- Mortgage paperwork and payments
- Loan documents
- IRA contributions
- Annual retirement and investment statements
- Tax returns and paperwork relating to taxes
- Pension plan documents
- Certificates for birth, adoption, marriage, divorce and death
- Deeds, trusts and wills
- Medical and prescription records
- Active life insurance policies
- Military discharge records
- Instruction books for appliances and electronics

When Warranty Expires:
- Bills and checks or credit card receipts for payment of item as well as the warranty itself

After 7 Years:
- Checks for charitable donations, tax payments and receipts for other tax-deductible expenses

After 1 Year:
- Cancelled checks (but see 7 years above)
- Paycheck stubs
- Utility bills
- Medical bills
- Bank statements (unless they support tax returns)
- Inactive insurance policies
- Other paid bills

After Receipt of Annual Statement or W2:
- Monthly retirement and investment statements

After 5 days:
- Credit card statement unless needed for tax purposes

After Receipt of Monthly Statement:
- Credit card receipts
- ATM and bank deposit receipts

Immediately:
- Unless listed above, anything that shows:
    Social security number
    Birth date
    Your signature
    Account numbers*
    Passwords*
    Pin numbers*
- Used airline tickets
- Preapproved credit card applications
- Expired driver's licenses, medical data and passports
- Unneeded copies of documents listed in the "Never" paragraph above

*Of course, you'll have this information recorded in a secure place.

Appendix B
Organizations that Accept a Variety of Items

Here's a list of websites with a brief description of what the organizations do (their programs and/or what they support). Note carefully whether the suffix is ".org" or ".com" as sometimes there are two different organizations. And websites come and go, so if the one shown doesn't work, Google just the organization for additional information.

Big Brothers/Big Sisters
>The world's largest one-on-one youth mentoring program.
>
>Accepts: clothing, exercise equipment, furniture, office supplies, and vehicles of all kinds including cars, trucks, motor homes, boats and even airplanes.

>### www.bbbs.org

>Click on (1) "Donate," (2) "Other Ways to Donate," and (3) "Learn More" (in the "Cars for Kids' Sake" section).

Goodwill Industries
>Using proceeds generated from donations sold in their stores, Goodwill provides job training for people who are looking for work or for a better job.
>
>Accepts: clothing, electrical and battery-operated items, children's games and toys and possibly vehicles and technology (including cell phones, computers, scanners, printers and software).

>### www.goodwill.org

ReUse Development Corporation (REDO)
>A non-profit filling the informational void to redistribute materials from those who no longer need items to those who can use them. Provides education, training and technical assistance to start-up reuse programs.
>
>Accepts: building materials, electronics, furniture (home and office), and household materials.

>### www.loadingdock.org/redo

>On the Redo website, click on "Find a Reuse Center."

Salvation Army

Disaster relief; helps with missing persons, conducts drug and alcohol rehabilitation programs, and facilitates programs that help society, too numerous to list here.

Accepts: airline miles, books, clothing, electronics, furniture, household goods, sporting equipment and vehicles.

www.salvationarmyusa.org

National Coalition for the Homeless

Works to meet the immediate needs of people who are currently experiencing homelessness or who are at risk of becoming so.

Accepts: clean clothing for current season; household goods including kitchen utensils and furniture, as well as games and toys; books; computers.

www.homelessshelterdirectory.org

Appendix C
Where to Donate Specific Items

Note carefully whether the suffix is ".org" or ".com" as sometimes there are two. And websites change, so if the one shown doesn't work, Google just the organization for additional information.

Children's Items

Room to Grow: baby furniture in excellent condition and new baby supplies for 1- 3 year old babies in poverty.

www.roomtogrow.org

Click on "baby supplies."

Project Night Night: kids' books, baby blankets and stuffed animals for homeless children.

www.projectnightnight.org

Shoes That Fit: shoes – suitable for school for children in need in the U.S.

www.shoesthatfit.org

Click on "Our Programs" and then "Schools We Help."

Stuffed Animals for Emergencies: stuffed animals - gently used, for kids in fires, accidents, neglected or abused, or impacted by tornadoes, floods and hurricanes.

www.stuffedanimalsforemergencies.org

Clothes

Career Gear: gives business attire for disconnected and underserved men – including suits, blazers, shoes, shirts, etc.; also men's toiletries when an interview is obtained.

www.careergear.org

Patagonia's Common Threads Garment Recycling: will recycle Capilene baselayer, Patagonia fleece, Polartec fleece (from any maker) and Patagonia cotton T-shirts into new clothing.

www.patagonia.com

Click on Repairs and Returns, and the fourth item down is "How To Recycle Patagonia Garments."

DonateMyDress: prom and Sweet 16 dresses for girls who cannot afford them.

www.donatemydress.org

Dress for Success: gives suits and accessories to disadvantaged women when an interview is obtained.

www.dressforsuccess.org

From this home page, click on "Support DFS," "Donate," and "Clothing" to find out what is needed. And again on the home page, click on "Locations" to know the affiliate nearest you.

Brides Against Breast Cancer: sells donated items and proceeds to make wishes and dreams come true for women and men who are losing their fight against breast cancer.
Accepts: Wedding gowns, slips, veils; diamonds; estate jewelry

www.bridesagainstbreastcancer.org/#donategown

Soles4Souls: Coordinated relief efforts for victims of Hurricanes Katrina and Rita and the Asian tsunami to provide shoes to the needy in the U.S. and over 100 countries.

www.soles4souls.org

Educational Materials

Books For Africa: has shipped over 20 million books to 45 countries. Books less than 15 years old - for all school grades.

Global Literacy Project: books – new and barely used for Africa, Asia and the Caribbean. Check their donation guidelines.

www.glpinc.org

Mr. Holland's Opus Foundation: musical instruments for school and after-school music programs that lack resources.

www.mhopus.org

In lower right panel, click on "Find out how."

Artists Working in Education: Provides children in Milwaukee area with art supplies and arts enrichment programs.

www.awe-inc.org

Home Stuff

Pets911: soft blankets, towels and linens (used in cages) at an animal shelter.

www.pets911.com

Google a website to find a shelter near you.

Habitat ReStores: sells merchandise at deep discount and proceeds go to Habitat For Humanity.

Accepts: building materials, accessories, appliances

www.habitat.org

To find a Resale outlet, click on (1) "Shop," (2) "Restore® Resale Outlets," (3) "Restore® Resale Outlets" (again, at bottom of page), and (4) "United States."

Furniture Bank Assn. of North America:
Furniture, beds, couches, dining room tables, and other furnishings for victims of natural disasters, those below the poverty line, and battered women and children in retreat.

www.nationalfurniturebank.org

For the bank closest to you click on "List of Furniture Banks" in left panel.

Magazines

Your local hospitals, women's shelters or retirement homes.

Personal

Unite for Sight: new sunglasses and prescription eyeglasses for the world's poorest people.

www.uniteforsight.org

Click on "Donate Now" on the extreme right of the top ribbon. Then either "Donate Eye Equipment" or "Donate Eyeglasses" in the left panel.

Give the Gift of Sight: cleans, repairs, classifies and delivers prescription or non-prescription eye and sunglasses in the U.S., South Africa and Central and South American countries.

www.givethegiftofsight.org

From their website: "Drop off your old eyeglasses or sunglasses at any LensCrafters, Pearle Vision, Sears Optical, Target Optical or Sunglass Hut store, or Lions club to help someone in a developing country experience a brighter future. We will clean, repair and classify your glasses by prescription, then personally deliver them on Give the Gift of Sight international optical missions."

New Eyes for the Needy: recycles donated eyeglasses for indigent children and buys new eyeglasses for poor children in the U.S.
Accepts: hearing aids, gold, silverware and giftware

www.neweyesfortheneedy.org

Lion's Clubs: disaster relief; provides service in communities of need in the U.S. and worldwide. Eyeglasses and hearing aids.
Accepts: eyeglasses and hearing aids

www.lionsclubs.org

For eyeglasses: enter "Donate Eyeglasses" in search box in upper right. In the list of articles that appear, click on "Donate Glasses – Lions Clubs – How You Can Help."
For hearing aids: Enter "donate hearing aids" in the search box in the upper right. In the list of articles that appear, click on "Donate Used Hearing Aids | Lions Hearing Aid…" to find a recycling center near you.

Starkey Hearing Foundation: delivers more than 50,000 hearing aids annually to countries from the U.S. to Vietnam.

www.sotheworldmayhear.org

Click on "Programs," and then "Hearing Aid Recycling."

Sports Clothing and Equipment

One World Running: athletic shoes – new and near-new sent to people in the U.S. and worldwide.

www.oneworldrunning.com

Then click on "Drop Off Locations" on ribbon at the top.

Nike's Reuse-A-Shoe: recycles any brand into soccer and football fields; and basketball and tennis courts. Athletic only, no metal or cleats.

www.nikereuseashoe.com

Click on "Get Involved." To print out a mailing label, click on "Individual Shoe Recycling." To locate a close drop off point click on "Drop Off Locations," fill in country and zip code, and click on "Find Locations."

Sports Gift: sports equipment and uniforms; coaching supplies for impoverished kids in community sports programs world-wide. Requested items only but their list, shown on their website, is quite extensive.

www.sportsgift.org

Click on "Collection Programs" and then, "Used Sports Items."

Technology: Cell and Wireless Phones

National Coalition Against Domestic Violence: to fund mission of ending violence in the home.

www.ncadv.org

Click on "Donate A Phone" in left panel.

Phones4Charity: refurbished phones sent to emerging countries and areas in U.S. for purposes of safety and communication.

www.phones4charity.org

Click on "Donate a Phone."

Cell Phones For Soldiers: to purchase calling cards for soldiers.

www.cellphonesforsoldiers.com

Technology: Computers, Printers and Software

World Computer Exchange: sends computers to kids in 68 countries; keeps computers out of landfills.

www.worldcomputerexchange.org

Click on "Support WCE" on ribbon and then "Donate Computers."

National Cristina Foundation: matches students at risk, the disabled and the underprivileged with hardware, software and training; has partner organizations for local donation.

www.cristina.org

Click on "Donate Now," and enter your zip code in the brown box to find out local organizations, and what is needed.

Technology: DVDs

Kid Flicks: has created over 500 movie libraries for children in hospitals; or donate directly to your local children's hospital.

www.kidflicks.org

Technology: Video Games and Systems

Get-Well Games Foundation: video game and game systems for children's hospitals in U.S.

www.get-well-gamers.org

Gamers Outreach: handheld electronic games for hospital patients and U.S. troops serving overseas.

www.gamersoutreach.org

Click on "Donate."

Vehicles: Cars, Trucks and Boats – even if not working

Cars For Kids: provides a second chance for at-risk kids through one-on-one education and training.

www.kars4kids.org

National Coalition Against Domestic Violence: proceeds used to support programs.

www.ncadv.org

Click on "Please Give" in the left panel.

Big Brothers and Big Sisters: the world's largest one-on-one youth mentoring program.

www.bbbs.org

Click on "Donate" and then "Other Ways to Donate."

Habitat for Humanity: builds and rehabs houses for people in need.

www.habitat.org

American Diabetes Association: works to prevent and cure diabetes and to improve the lives of all people affected by diabetes.

www.diabetes.org

1-800-Charity Cars: gives vehicles to struggling families willing to work.

www.800charitycars.org

Appendix 1
Creating Tables and Saving Time: Word® 2004 For Macs

My curiosity to learn new functions of Word® over the years yielded a couple of tricks that I now use constantly. First, I learned how to create a table, and then how to find a word or phrase quickly or sort information within the table. The "Header and Footer" function will insert the date and time, file name, and page numbers on every page in a document. I believe you will find all this helpful, too.

Creating a Table of Columns and Rows – To Organize Information Better

1. Click on the **Blue "W" icon** at the bottom of the screen. If not there, get some help as described in Chapter 28. If a blank page is not displayed, click on **FILE > NEW BLANK DOCUMENT.**

2. Click on **TABLE > INSERT > TABLE.**

3. Choose columns and rows wanted from drop down box. Click on **OK.**

4. To change the number of rows or columns, highlight the area, click on **TABLE > INSERT (or DELETE),** and choose desired action.

   Instructions on how to highlight are found in Chapter 28, but note paragraph 3e in the section on "Sorting Items in a Table" found below.

   Column width and row height are changed by placing cursor on appropriate line, and when a double-headed arrow appears (<u>left and right</u> for column width and <u>up and down</u> for row height), hold the mouse down and move in the appropriate direction.

Rows can be added quickly by clicking inside any cell and holding down the **TAB** key.

<u>To Copy and Paste – To Save Time</u>

1. Click to the left of the first letter of the text to be copied, and highlight the area.

   The use of the word "text" includes letters, digits, tables, or whatever.

2. Click on **EDIT > COPY.**

3. Click on the area where the information <u>is</u> to appear.

4. Click on **EDIT > PASTE** or **PASTE COLUMNS.**

It's that easy!

<u>Sorting Items in a Table – To Rearrange Information</u>
Information is entered into a table arbitrarily, and a list of cardboard boxes containing file folders might look like this:

Box #	Subject
Box 1	2008 Investment Account Reports
Box 1	56 Main Street, Providence - Purchase
Box 2	Marriage Certificate for Us
Box 3	364 Jones Avenue, Wakefield - Sale
Box 4	Divorce - Mary - 1998
Box 4	Marriage - Mary - 1985
Box 5	London Trip - Fall 2010
Box 5	New York City Trip - Spring 2011
Box 6	2006 Budget
Box 6	2008 Federal and State Tax Returns

Table #1

1. Click to the left of the first letter of the text to be sorted, and highlight the area.

2. Click on **TABLE > SORT**

3. In "Sort" drop down box:

    a. Choose **PRIMARY**[10] sort in "Sort by" box. In Table #2 (below), "Subject" or "Column 2" is the primary sort.

    b. Determine **SECONDARY** sort in "Then by" box. In Table #2 (below), "Box #" or "Column 1" is the secondary sort.

    c. Select **Text, Number** or **Date** in "Type" box.

    "Text" will sort alphabetically on the first digit. Thus, numbers precede letters. "Numbers" arranges items by value, and "Date" organizes information chronologically.

    "Text" was used for both columns in Table #2.

    d. Indicate **Ascending** (A-Z) or **Descending** (Z-A).

    "Ascending" was used for both columns in Table #2.

    e. In the "My list has" section, click on the **Header row** or **No header row** button. This will define the highlighted area.

    A "header row" is the heading (or description) of a column. In the tables shown, the header row displays "Box #" and "Subject." If the "Header row" button is filled in, the "Sort by" and "Then by" boxes will show "Box #" and "Subject" respectively as sorting criteria. If the "No header row" is indicated, these boxes will display "Column 1" and "Column 2."

10. The primary sort is the first order in which information will be listed. For example, a list of cities and their street names would place all cities together, and then streets within that city would be shown alphabetically. The city is the primary sort and streets the secondary sort.

f. Click on **OK.**

And the table becomes:

Box #	Subject
Box 6	2006 Budget
Box 6	2008 Federal and State Tax Returns
Box 1	2008 Investment Account Reports
Box 3	364 Jones Avenue, Wakefield - Sale
Box 1	56 Main Street, Providence - Purchase
Box 4	Divorce - Mary - 1998
Box 5	London Trip - Fall 2010
Box 2	Marriage Certificate for Us
Box 4	Marriage - Mary - 1985
Box 5	New York City Trip - Spring 2011

Table #2

Note that since "Text" was used in paragraph 3c above, items are alphabetical in the "Subject" column and thus "2006" is shown before "56."

From this, I learned that records for 2008 were in different boxes and records on marriage were too.

The SORT function is very handy because my own "archives" contain too many files in boxes in the cellar. Someday someone will bless me (I hope) or curse me for keeping all this stuff.

The "FIND" Function – To Locate Information

1. Click to the left of the first letter or digit where the search will start.

2. Click on **EDIT > FIND.**

3. In the box that pops up, **type the words or digits** to be found (criteria).

4. Click on **FIND NEXT.**

The first match will be highlighted and then wait. When the **FIND NEXT** or **RETURN** button is clicked again, the cursor will hopscotch to the next place in the document that matches your criteria, until a box appears that "Word has finished searching the document."

5. Click on **YES > OK > CANCEL** or **NO > CANCEL.**

Bingo! The information has been located quickly.

The "Header or Footer" Function – To Show File Name, Date/Time and Page Numbers

1. Click on **VIEW > HEADER and FOOTER.**

   The cursor will appear in the header. Scroll down and click on footer if desired. Both will be closed when **CLOSE** is clicked.

2. On the horizontal bar that appears and starts with "Auto Text,"

   a. For Date: click on the icon that looks like **TWO CALENDAR PAGES.**

   b. For Time: click on the **CLOCK.**

   c. For the Location of the File on Your Computer: click on **AUTOTEXT > FILENAME AND PATH.**

   d. For Page Numbers: **AUTOTEXT > PAGE X OF Y.**

   e. Click on **CLOSE.**

It's all pretty nifty.

So much for the mechanics of creating and using tables as well as saving time.

Appendix 2
Creating Tables and Saving Time: Word® 2008 For Macs

My curiosity to learn new functions of Word® over the years yielded a couple of tricks that I now use constantly. First, I learned how to create a table, and then how to find a word or phrase quickly or sort information within the table. The "Header and Footer" function will insert the date and time, file name, and page numbers on every page in a document. I know you will find all this helpful, too.

Creating a Table of Columns and Rows – To Organize Information Better

1. Click on the **Blue "W" icon** at the bottom or side of the screen.

   If not there, get some help as described in Chapter 28. If a blank page is not displayed, click on **FILE > NEW BLANK DOCUMENT.**

2. Click on **TABLE > INSERT > TABLE.**

3. Choose columns and rows wanted from drop down box. Click on **OK.**

4. To change the number of rows or columns, highlight the area, click on **TABLE > INSERT (or DELETE)**, and choose desired action.

   Instructions on how to highlight are found in Chapter 28, but note paragraph 3e in the section on "Sorting Items in a Table" found below.

   Column width and row height are changed by placing cursor on appropriate line, and when a double-headed arrow appears (left and right for column width and up and down for row height), hold the mouse down and move in the appropriate direction.

Rows can be added quickly by clicking inside any cell and holding down the **TAB** key.

To Copy and Paste – To Save Time

1. Click to the left of the first letter of the text to be copied, and highlight the area.

   The use of the word "text" includes letters, digits, tables or whatever.

2. Click on **EDIT > COPY**.

3. Click on the area where the information is to appear.

4. Click on **EDIT > PASTE** or **PASTE COLUMNS**.

It's that easy!

Sorting Items in a Table – To Rearrange Information

Information is entered into a table arbitrarily, and a list of cardboard boxes containing file folders might look like this:

Box #	Subject
Box 1	2008 Investment Account Reports
Box 1	56 Main Street, Providence - Purchase
Box 2	Marriage Certificate for Us
Box 3	364 Jones Avenue, Wakefield - Sale
Box 4	Divorce - Mary - 1998
Box 4	Marriage - Mary - 1985
Box 5	London Trip - Fall 2010
Box 5	New York City Trip - Spring 2011
Box 6	2006 Budget
Box 6	2008 Federal and State Tax Returns

Table #1

1. Click to the left of the first letter of the text to be sorted, and highlight the area.

2. Click on **TABLE > SORT.**

3. In "Sort" drop down box:

   a. Choose **PRIMARY**[10] sort in "Sort by" box. In Table #2 (below), "Subject" or "Column 2" is the primary sort.

   b. Determine **SECONDARY** sort in "Then by" box. In Table #2 (below), "Box #" or "Column 1" is the secondary sort.

   c. Select **Text, Number** or **Date** in "Type" box.

   "Text" will sort alphabetically on the first digit. Thus, numbers precede letters. "Numbers" arranges items by value, and "Date" organizes information chronologically.

   "Text" was used for both columns in Table #2.

   d. Indicate **Ascending** (A-Z) or **Descending** (Z-A).

   "Ascending" was used for both columns in Table #2.

   e. In the "My list has" section, click on the **Header row** or **No header row** button. This will define the highlighted area.

   A "header row" is the heading (or description) of a column. In the tables shown, the header row displays "Box #" and "Subject." If the "Header row" button is filled in, the "Sort

---

10. The primary sort is the first order in which information will be listed. For example, a list of cities and their street names would place all cities together, and then streets within that city would be shown alphabetically. The city is the primary sort and streets the secondary sort.

by" and "Then by" boxes will show "Box #" and
"Subject" respectively as sorting criteria. If the
"No header row" is indicated, these boxes will
display "Column 1" and "Column 2."

f. Click on **OK**.

And the table becomes:

Box #	Subject
Box 6	2006 Budget
Box 6	2008 Federal and State Tax Returns
Box 1	2008 Investment Account Reports
Box 3	364 Jones Avenue, Wakefield - Sale
Box 1	56 Main Street, Providence - Purchase
Box 4	Divorce - Mary - 1998
Box 5	London Trip - Fall 2010
Box 2	Marriage Certificate for Us
Box 4	Marriage - Mary - 1985
Box 5	New York City Trip - Spring 2011

Table #2

Note that since "Text" was used in paragraph 3c above, items are
alphabetical in the "Subject" column and thus "2006" is shown before
"56".

From this, I learned that records for 2008 were in different boxes and
records on marriage were too.

The SORT function is very handy because my own "archives" contain
too many files in 27 boxes in the cellar. Someday someone will bless
me (I hope) or curse me for keeping all this stuff.

The "FIND" Function – To Locate Information

1. Click to the left of the first letter or digit where the
   search will start.

2. Click on **EDIT > FIND.**

3. In the box that pops up, **type the words or digits to**

185

be found (criteria).

4. Click on **FIND NEXT.**

The first match will be highlighted and then wait. When the **FIND NEXT** or **RETURN** button is clicked again, the cursor will hopscotch to the next place in the document that matches your criteria, until a box appears that "Word has finished searching the document."

5. Click on **OK > CANCEL.**

Bingo! The information has been located quickly.

The "Header or Footer" Function – To Show File Name, Date/Time and Page Numbers

1. Click on **VIEW > HEADER and FOOTER.**

The cursor will appear in the header. Scroll down and click on footer if desired. Both will be closed when **CLOSE** is clicked.

2. For Location of File on Your Computer: **INSERT > AUTOTEXT > FILENAME and PATH.**

3. For Date and Time: **INSERT > DATE and TIME**; Choose format, click on **UPDATE AUTOMATICALLY** if desired > **OK.**

4. For Page X of Y: **INSERT > AUTOTEXT > PAGE X of Y.**

5. Click on **CLOSE.**

It's all pretty nifty.

So much for the mechanics of creating and using tables as well as saving time.

Appendix 3
Creating Tables and Saving Time: Word® 2011 For Macs

My curiosity to learn new functions of Word® over the years yielded a couple of tricks that I now use constantly. First, I learned how to create a table, and then how to find a word or phrase quickly or sort information within the table. The "Header and Footer" function will insert the date and time, file name, and page numbers on every page in a document. I believe you will find all this helpful, too.

Creating a Table of Columns and Rows – To Organize Information Better

1. Click on the **Blue "W" icon** at the bottom or side of the screen.

   If not there, get some help as described in Chapter 28. If a blank page is not displayed, click on **FILE > NEW BLANK DOCUMENT.**

2. Click on **TABLE > INSERT > TABLE.**

3. **Choose** columns and rows wanted from drop down box. Click on **OK.**

4. To change the number of rows or columns, highlight the area, click on **TABLE > INSERT (or DELETE),** and choose desired action.

   Instructions on how to highlight are found in Chapter 28, but note paragraph 3e in the section on "Sorting Items in a Table" found below.

Column width and row height are changed by placing cursor on appropriate line, and when a double-headed arrow appears (<u>left and right</u> for column width and <u>up and down</u> for row height), hold the mouse down and move in the appropriate direction.

Rows can be added quickly by clicking inside any cell and holding down the **TAB** key.

To Copy and Paste – To Save Time

1. Click to the left of the first letter of the text to be copied, and highlight the area.

   The use of the word "text" includes letters, digits, tables, or whatever.

2. Click on **EDIT > COPY**.

3. Click on the area where the information <u>is</u> to appear.

4. Click on **EDIT > PASTE** or **PASTE COLUMNS**.

It's that easy!

Sorting Items in a Table – To Rearrange Information

Information is entered into a table arbitrarily, and a list of cardboard boxes containing file folders might look like this:

Box #	Subject
Box 1	2008 Investment Account Reports
Box 1	56 Main Street, Providence - Purchase
Box 2	Marriage Certificate for Us
Box 3	364 Jones Avenue, Wakefield - Sale
Box 4	Divorce - Mary - 1998
Box 4	Marriage - Mary - 1985
Box 5	London Trip - Fall 2010
Box 5	New York City Trip - Spring 2011
Box 6	2006 Budget
Box 6	2008 Federal and State Tax Returns

Table #1

1. Click to the left of the first letter of the text to be sorted, and highlight the area.

2. Click on TABLE > SORT.

3. In "Sort" drop down box:

   a. Choose **PRIMARY**[10] sort in "Sort by" box. In Table #2 (below), "Subject" or "Column 2" is the primary sort.

   b. Determine **SECONDARY** sort in "Then by" box. In Table #2 (below), "Box #" or "Column 1" is the secondary sort.

   c. Select **Text, Number** or **Date** in "Type" box.

   "Text" will sort alphabetically on the first digit. Thus, numbers precede letters. "Numbers" arranges items by value, and "Date" organizes information chronologically.

   "Text" was used for both columns in Table #2.

   d. Indicate **Ascending** (A-Z) or **Descending** (Z-A).

   "Ascending" was used for both columns in Table #2.

   e. In the "My list has" section, click on the **Header row** or **No header** row button. This will define the highlighted area.

   A "header row" is the heading (or description) of a column. In the tables shown, the header row displays "Box #" and "Subject." If the "Header row" button is filled in, the "Sort by" and "Then by" boxes will show "Box #" and "Subject" respectively as sorting criteria. If the

10. The primary sort is the first order in which information will be listed. For example, a list of cities and their street names would place all cities together, and then streets within that city would be shown alphabetically. The city is the primary sort and streets the secondary sort.

"No header row" is indicated, these boxes will display "Column 1" and "Column 2."

f. Click on **OK.**

And the table becomes:

Box #	Subject
Box 6	2006 Budget
Box 6	2008 Federal and State Tax Returns
Box 1	2008 Investment Account Reports
Box 3	364 Jones Avenue, Wakefield - Sale
Box 1	56 Main Street, Providence - Purchase
Box 4	Divorce - Mary - 1998
Box 5	London Trip - Fall 2010
Box 2	Marriage Certificate for Us
Box 4	Marriage - Mary - 1985
Box 5	New York City Trip - Spring 2011

Table #2

Note that since "Text" was used in paragraph 3c above, items are alphabetical in the "Subject" column and thus "2006" is shown before "56."

From this, I learned that records for 2008 were in different boxes and records on marriage were too.

The SORT function is very handy because my own "archives" contain too many files in boxes in the cellar. Someday someone will bless me (I hope) or curse me for keeping all this stuff.

The "FIND" Function – To Locate Information

1. Click to the left of the first letter or digit where the search will start.

2. Click on **EDIT > FIND > ADVANCED FIND AND REPLACE.**

3. In the box that pops up, **type the words or digits** to be found (criteria).

4. Click on **FIND NEXT.**

The first match will be highlighted and then wait. When the **FIND NEXT** or **RETURN** button is clicked again, the cursor will hopscotch to the next place in the document that matches your criteria, until a box appears that "Word has finished searching the document."

5. Click on **YES > OK** or **NO > CANCEL**.

when the balance of the file has been searched.

Bingo! The information has been located quickly.

The "Header or Footer" Function – To Show File Name, Date/Time and Page Numbers

1. Click on **VIEW > HEADER or FOOTER.**

The cursor will appear in the header. Scroll down and click on footer if desired. Both will be closed when **CLOSE** is clicked.

2. For Location of File on Your Computer: **INSERT > AUTOTEXT > FILENAME and PATH > OK.**

3. For Date and Time: **INSERT > DATE and TIME > OK.**

In the **DATE and TIME** drop down box, choose style, and if wanted, click on **UPDATE AUTOMATICALLY.**

4. For Page X of Y: **INSERT > AUTOTEXT > PAGE X of Y**.

5. Click on **CLOSE.**

It's all pretty nifty.

So much for all the mechanics of creating and using tables as well as saving time.

Appendix 4
Creating Tables and Saving Time: Word® 2003 For PCs

My curiosity to learn new functions of Word® over the years yielded a couple of tricks that I now use constantly. First, I learned how to create a table, and then how to find a word or phrase quickly or sort information within the table. The "Header and Footer" function will insert the date and time, file name, and page numbers on every page in a document. I believe you will find all this helpful, too.

Creating a Table of Columns and Rows – To Organize Information Better

1. Click on the **Blue "W" icon** at the bottom or side of the screen.

   If not there, get some help as described in Chapter 28. If a blank page is not displayed, click on **FILE > NEW BLANK DOCUMENT.**

2. Click on **TABLE > INSERT > TABLE.**

3. Choose columns and rows wanted from drop down box. Click on **OK.**

4. To change the number of rows or columns, highlight the area, click on **TABLE > INSERT (or DELETE),** and choose desired action.

   Instructions on how to highlight are found in Chapter 28, but note paragraph 3e in the section on "Sorting Items in a Table" found below.

   Column width and row height are changed by placing cursor on appropriate line, and when a double-headed arrow appears (<u>left and right</u> for column width and <u>up and down</u> for row height), hold the mouse down and move in the appropriate direction.

Rows can be added quickly by clicking inside any cell and holding down the **TAB** key.

To Copy and Paste – To Save Time

1. Click to the left of the first letter of the text to be copied, and highlight the area.

    The use of the word "text" includes letters, digits tables, or whatever.

2. Click on **EDIT > COPY.**

3. Click on the area where the information <u>is</u> to appear.

4. Click on **EDIT > PASTE or PASTE CELLS.**

It's that easy!

Sorting Items in a Table – To Rearrange Information

Information is entered into a table arbitrarily, and a list of cardboard boxes containing file folders might look like this:

Box #	Subject
Box 1	2008 Investment Account Reports
Box 1	56 Main Street, Providence - Purchase
Box 2	Marriage Certificate for Us
Box 3	364 Jones Avenue, Wakefield - Sale
Box 4	Divorce - Mary - 1998
Box 4	Marriage - Mary - 1985
Box 5	London Trip - Fall 2010
Box 5	New York City Trip - Spring 2011
Box 6	2006 Budget
Box 6	2008 Federal and State Tax Returns

Table #1

1. Click to the left of the first letter of the text to be sorted, and highlight the area.

2. Click on **TABLE** > **SORT**.

3. In "Sort" drop down box:

   a. Choose **PRIMARY**[10] sort in "Sort by" box. In Table #2 (below), "Subject" or Column 2" is the primary sort.

   b. Determine **SECONDARY** sort in "Then by" box.

   In Table #2 (below), "Box #" or "Column 1" is the secondary sort.

   c. Select **Text, Number** or **Date** in "Type" box.

   "Text" will sort alphabetically on the first digit. Thus, numbers precede letters. "Numbers" arranges items by value, and "Date" organizes information chronologically.

   "Text" was used for both columns in Table #2.

   d. Indicate **Ascending** (A-Z) or **Descending** (Z-A).

   "Ascending" was used for both columns in Table #2.

   e. In the "My list has" section, click the **Header row** or **No header row** button. This will define the highlighted area.

   A "header row" is the heading (or description) of a column. In the tables shown, the header row displays "Box #" and "Subject." If the "Header row" button is filled in, the "Sort by" and "Then by" boxes will show "Box #" and "Subject" respectively as sorting criteria. If the

---

10. The primary sort is the first order in which information will be listed. For example, a list of cities and their street names would place all cities together, and then streets within that city would be shown alphabetically. The city is the primary sort and streets the secondary sort.

"No header row" is indicated, these boxes will display "Column 1" and "Column 2."

    f. Click on **OK.**

And the table becomes:

Box #	Subject
Box 6	2006 Budget
Box 6	2008 Federal and State Tax Returns
Box 1	2008 Investment Account Reports
Box 3	364 Jones Avenue, Wakefield - Sale
Box 1	56 Main Street, Providence - Purchase
Box 4	Divorce - Mary - 1998
Box 5	London Trip - Fall 2010
Box 2	Marriage Certificate for Us
Box 4	Marriage - Mary - 1985
Box 5	New York City Trip - Spring 2011

Table #2

Note that since "Text" was used in paragraph 3c above, items are alphabetical in the "Subject" column and thus "2006" is shown before "56."

From this, I learned that records for 2008 were in different boxes and records on marriage were too.

The SORT function is very handy because my own "archives" contain too many files in boxes in the cellar. Someday someone will bless me (I hope) or curse me for keeping all this stuff.

The "FIND" Function – To Locate Information

    1. Click to the left of the first letter or digit where the search will start.

    2. Click on **EDIT > FIND.**

    3. In the box that pops up, **type the words or digits** to be found (criteria).

    4. Click on **FIND NEXT.**

The first match will be highlighted and then wait. When the **FIND NEXT** or **RETURN** button is clicked again, the cursor will hopscotch to the next place in the document that matches your criteria, until a box appears that "Word has finished searching the document."

    5. Click on **OK > CANCEL.**

Bingo! The information has been located quickly.

The "Header or Footer" Function – To Show File Name, Date/Time and Page Numbers

    1. Click on **VIEW > HEADER and FOOTER.**

The cursor will appear in the header. Scroll down and click on footer if desired. Both will be closed when **CLOSE** is clicked.

    2. On the horizontal bar that appears and starts with "Auto Text,"

        a. For Date: click on the icon that looks like **TWO CALENDAR PAGES.**

        b. For Time: click on the **CLOCK.**

        c. For the Location of the File on Your Computer: click **AUTOTEXT > FILENAME AND PATH.**

        d. For Page Numbers: **AUTOTEXT > PAGE X of Y.**

        e. Click on **CLOSE**

It's all pretty nifty.

So much for the mechanics of creating and using tables as well as saving time.

Appendix 5
Creating Tables and Saving Time: Word® 2007 For PCs

My curiosity to learn new functions of Word® over the years yielded a couple of tricks that I now use constantly. First, I learned how to create a table, and then how to find a word or phrase quickly or sort information within the table. The "Header and Footer" function will insert the date and time, file name, and page numbers on every page in a document. I believe you will find all this helpful, too.

Creating a Table of Columns and Rows – To Organize Information Better

1. Click on the **Blue "W"** icon at the bottom or side of the computer screen.

   If not there, get some help as described in Chapter 28. If a blank page is not displayed, click on **FILE > NEW.**

2. Click on **INSERT > TABLE.**

3. Place mouse arrow on upper left box of squares, and **scroll** across and down from the upper left box until the desired columns and rows are highlighted. Click on lower right box.

4. Adding, Deleting and Adjusting the Size of Columns, Rows and the Entire Table:

   a. To add: **Highlight** area of change, click on **LAYOUT**, and in the "Rows and Columns" icon group, choose the addition wanted.

   Note: click on **LAYOUT** – not Page Layout.

Instructions on how to highlight are found in Chapter 28, but note paragraph 3e in the section on "Sorting Items in a Table" found below.

Rows can be added quickly by clicking inside any cell and holding down the TAB key.

b. <u>To delete:</u> Highlight area to be deleted, click on **LAYOUT > DELETE**, and select changes in drop down box.

c. <u>To adjust size:</u> Place cursor on appropriate line, and when two arrows appear (<u>left and right</u> for column width and <u>up and down</u> for row height), hold mouse down and move in the appropriate direction.

To Copy and Paste – To Save Time

1. Click to the left of the first letter of the text to be copied, and highlight the area.

The use of the word "text" includes letters, digits, tables, or whatever.

2. Click on **HOME > COPY** (the icon of **TWO PAGES** on extreme left).

3. Click on the area where the information <u>is</u> to appear.

4. Click on **HOME > PASTE.**

It's that easy!

Sorting Items in a Table – To Rearrange Information

Information is entered line by line into a chart, and a list of boxes containing file folders might look like this:

Box #	Subject
Box 1	2008 Investment Account Reports
Box 1	56 Main Street, Providence - Purchase
Box 2	Marriage Certificate for Us
Box 3	364 Jones Avenue, Wakefield - Sale
Box 4	Divorce - Mary - 1998
Box 4	Marriage - Mary - 1985
Box 5	London Trip - Fall 2010
Box 5	New York City Trip - Spring 2011
Box 6	2006 Budget
Box 6	2008 Federal and State Tax Returns

Table #1

1. Highlight area to be sorted.

2. Click on **LAYOUT > SORT.**

3. In "Sort" drop down box:

    a. Choose **PRIMARY**[10] sort in "Sort by" box.

    In Table #2 (below), "Subject" or "Column 2" is the primary sort.

    b. Determine **SECONDARY** sort in "Then by" box.

    In Table #2 (below), "Box #" or "Column 1" is the secondary sort.

    c. Select **Text, Number** or **Date** in "Type" box.

    "Text" will sort alphabetically on the first digit. Thus, numbers precede letters. "Numbers" arranges items by value, and "Date" organizes information chronologically.

10. The primary sort is the first order in which information will be listed. For example, a list of cities and their street names would place all cities together, and then streets within that city would be shown alphabetically. The city is the primary sort and streets the secondary sort.

"Text" was used for both columns in Table #2.

d. Indicate **Ascending (A-Z)** or **Descending (Z-A)**.

Ascending was used in both columns in Table #2.

e. In the "My List has" section, select the **Header row** or **No header row** button. This will define the highlighted area.

A "header row" is the heading (or description) of a column. In the tables shown, the header row displays "Box #" and "Subject." If the "Header row" button is filled in, the "Sort by" and "Then by" boxes will show "Box #" and "Subject" respectively as sorting criteria. If the "No header row" is indicated, these boxes will display "Column 1" and "Column 2."

f. Click on **OK.**

And the table becomes:

Box #	Subject
Box 6	2006 Budget
Box 6	2008 Federal and State Tax Returns
Box 1	2008 Investment Account Reports
Box 3	364 Jones Avenue, Wakefield - Sale
Box 1	56 Main Street, Providence - Purchase
Box 4	Divorce - Mary - 1998
Box 5	London Trip - Fall 2010
Box 2	Marriage Certificate for Us
Box 4	Marriage - Mary - 1985
Box 5	New York City Trip - Spring 2011

Table #2

Note that since "Text" was used in paragraph 3c above, items are alphabetical in the "Subject" column and thus "2006" is shown before "56."

From this, I learned that records for 2008 were in different boxes and records on marriage were too.

The SORT function is very handy because my own "archives" contain too many files in boxes in the cellar. Someday someone will bless me (I hope) or curse me for keeping all this stuff.

The "FIND" Function – To Locate Information

1. Click to the left of the first letter or digit where the search will start.

2. Click on **HOME> FIND** on the extreme right.

3. In the window that pops up, type the information to be found (criteria).

4. Click on **FIND NEXT.**

   The first match will be highlighted and then wait. When the **FIND NEXT** or **RETURN** button is clicked again, the cursor will hopscotch to the next place in the document that matches your criteria, until a box appears that "Word has finished searching the document."

5. Click on **YES> OK > CANCEL** or **NO>CANCEL.**

Bingo! The information has been located quickly.

The "Header or Footer" Function – To Show File Name, Date/Time and Page Numbers

1. To Create Header or Footer:

   a. Click on **INSERT > HEADER** or **FOOTER.**

   b. In the "Built In" drop down box, select format wanted. Choose "Blank."

c. "[Type Text]" will appear. Enter text if desired or **DELETE** on the keyboard.

2. For Location of File on Your Computer:

a. Click on **DESIGN > QUICK PARTS > FIELD**.

b. Scroll down to and click on **FILENAME > ADD PATH TO FILENAME > OK**.

3. To Add Date and Time:

a. Click on **DESIGN > DATE AND TIME**.

b. Select style wanted and if desired, choose **UPDATE AUTOMATICALLY > OK**.

4. To Insert Page X of Y:

a. Click on **DESIGN > PAGE NUMBER**.

b. Choose **CURRENT POSITION**, and in drop down box on right, scroll down to and click on box that says **PAGE X of Y**.

Box will also show "1 of 1."

5. To Close Header or Footer:

Click on **DESIGN > CLOSE HEADER AND FOOTER**.

It's all pretty nifty.

So much for the mechanics of creating and using tables as well as saving time.

Appendix 6
Creating Tables and Saving Time: Word® 2010 For PCs

My curiosity to learn new functions of Word® over the years yielded a couple of tricks that I now use constantly. First, I learned how to create a table, and then how to find a word or phrase quickly or sort information within the table. The "Header and Footer" function will insert the date and time, file name, and page numbers on every page in a document. I believe you will find all this helpful, too.

Creating a Table of Columns and Rows – To Organize Information Better

1. Click on the **Blue "W"** icon at the bottom or side of the computer screen.

   If not there, get some help as described in Chapter 28. If a blank page is not displayed, click on **FILE > NEW.**

2. Click on **INSERT > TABLE.**

3. Place mouse arrow on upper left box of squares, and scroll across and down from the upper left box until the desired columns and rows are highlighted. Click on lower right box.

4. Adding, Deleting and Adjusting the Size of Columns, Rows and the Entire Table:

   a. To add: Highlight area of change, click on **LAY OUT**, and in the "Rows and Columns" icon group, choose the addition wanted.

   Note: click on **LAYOUT** – not **Page Layout**

Instructions on how to highlight are found in Chapter 28, but note paragraph 3e in the section on "Sorting Items in a Table" found below.

Rows can be added quickly by clicking inside any cell and holding down the **TAB** key.

b. <u>To delete:</u> highlight area to be deleted, click on **LAYOUT** > **DELETE**, and select changes in drop down box.

c. <u>To adjust size:</u> Place cursor on appropriate line, and when a double-headed arrow appears (<u>left and right</u> for column width and <u>up and down</u> for row height), hold the mouse down and move in the appropriate direction.

To Copy and Paste – To Save Time

1. Click to the left of the first letter of the text to be copied, and highlight the area.

   The use of the word "text" includes letters, digits, tables, or whatever.

2. Click on **HOME** > **COPY** (the icon of **TWO PAGES** on extreme left).

3. Click on the area where the information <u>is</u> to appear.

4. Click on **HOME** > **PASTE.**

It's that easy!

Sorting Items in a Table – To Rearrange Information

Information is entered line by line into a chart, and a list of boxes containing file folders might look like this:

Box #	Subject
Box 1	2008 Investment Account Reports
Box 1	56 Main Street, Providence - Purchase
Box 2	Marriage Certificate for Us
Box 3	364 Jones Avenue, Wakefield - Sale
Box 4	Divorce - Mary - 1998
Box 4	Marriage - Mary - 1985
Box 5	London Trip - Fall 2010
Box 5	New York City Trip - Spring 2011
Box 6	2006 Budget
Box 6	2008 Federal and State Tax Returns

Table #1

1. Highlight area to be sorted.

2. Click on **LAYOUT > SORT.**

3. In "Sort" drop down box:

    a. Choose **PRIMARY**[10] sort in "Sort by" box.

    In Table #2 (below), "Subject" or "Column 2" is the primary sort.

    b. Determine **SECONDARY** sort in "Then by" box.

    In Table #2 (below), "Box #" or "Column 1" is the secondary sort.

    c. Select **Text, Number** or **Date** in "Type" box.

    "Text" will sort alphabetically on the first digit. Thus, numbers precede letters. "Numbers" arranges items by value, and "Date" organizes information chronologically.

10. The primary sort is the first order in which information will be listed. For example, a list of cities and their street names would place all cities together, and then streets within that city would be shown alphabetically. The city is the primary sort and streets the secondary sort.

"Text" was used for both columns in Table #2.

d. Indicate **Ascending (A-Z) or Descending (Z-A).**

"Ascending" was used for both columns in Table #2.

e. In the "My list has" section, click on the **Header row** or **No header row** button. This will define the highlighted area.

A "header row" is the heading (or description) of a column. In the tables shown, the header row displays "Box #" and "Subject." If the "Header row" button is filled in, the "Sort by" and "Then by" boxes will show "Box #" and "Subject" respectively as sorting criteria. If the "No header row" is indicated, these boxes will display "Column 1" and "Column 2."

f. Click on **OK.**

And the table becomes:

Box #	Subject
Box 6	2006 Budget
Box 6	2008 Federal and State Tax Returns
Box 1	2008 Investment Account Reports
Box 3	364 Jones Avenue, Wakefield - Sale
Box 1	56 Main Street, Providence - Purchase
Box 4	Divorce - Mary - 1998
Box 5	London Trip - Fall 2010
Box 2	Marriage Certificate for Us
Box 4	Marriage - Mary - 1985
Box 5	New York City Trip - Spring 2011

Table #2

Note that since "Text" was used in paragraph 3c above, items are alphabetical in the "Subject" column and thus "2006" is shown before "56."

From this, I learned that records for 2008 were in different boxes and records on marriage were too.

The SORT function is very handy because my own "archives" contain too many files in boxes in the cellar. Someday someone will bless me (I hope) or curse me for keeping all this stuff.

The "FIND" Function – To Locate Information

1. Highlight area to be searched.

2. Click on **HOME > FIND** (on extreme right).

3. Enter the information to be found (criteria) in the "Search Document" box of the "Navigation" window.

4. When the various matches shown in the "Navigation" panel are clicked, the cursor will go to that place in the file where the criteria appear.

5. Click on the **X** on the "Navigation" panel to close it.

Bingo! The information has been located quickly.

The "Header or Footer" Function – To Show File Name, Date/Time and Page Numbers

1. To Create Header or Footer:

   a. Click on **INSERT > HEADER or FOOTER.**

   b. In the "Built In," drop down box, select format wanted. (Choose "Blank.")

   c. "[Type Text]" will appear. Enter **DELETE** on the keyboard and enter text, if desired.

2. For Location of File on Your Computer:

   a. Click on **DESIGN > QUICK PARTS > FIELD.**

b. Scroll down to and click on **FILENAME > ADD PATH TO FILENAME > OK.**

3. To Add Date and Time:

   a. Click on DESIGN > DATE AND TIME.

   b. Select style wanted and if desired, choose **UPDATE AUTOMATICALLY > OK.**

4. To Insert Page X of Y:

   a. Click on **DESIGN > PAGE NUMBER.**

   b. Choose **CURRENT POSITION**, and in drop down box on right, scroll down to and click on box that says **PAGE X of Y.**

   Box will also show "1 of 1."

5. To Close Header or Footer:

   Click on **DESIGN > CLOSE HEADER AND FOOTER.**

It's all pretty nifty.

So much for the mechanics of creating and using tables as well as saving time.

BONUS: Download the FREE companion app at www.MyFamilyRecordBook.com

About the Author

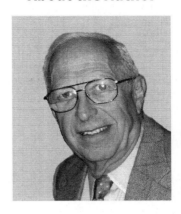

Harris "Hershey" Rosen, a graduate of Harvard, has focused on controlling chaos since 1954. First, as Financial Control Officer in the U.S. Army, where he received a Letter of Commendation for improvement to its worldwide accounting system. Next, on to satisfying everyone's sweet tooth, he ran a candy company for 40 years, developing a system for locating ANY item housed in five factories, covering 600,000 sq. ft. Following "retirement," Hershey went on to become a mediator and settled over 200 disputes for the State of Rhode Island and The Community Mediation Center of Rhode Island. He was also asked to team-teach management courses at the University of Rhode Island, where he enthusiastically challenged the text book with real-life experience, to the delight and edification of the students. Always passionate about assisting others, Hershey has been the director or trustee of numerous boards and organizations. He has most recently written *My Family Record Book* to help others protect their spouses (and families) from the intense stress that will occur if one does not share knowledge critical to a functioning home.

Hershey, who lives in Providence, Rhode Island, can now relax (ha!) with his beloved wife, Myrna, and enjoy visits with their combined five children and ten grandchildren. He may be reached at survivorinfo@aol.com.

INDEX

Made in the USA
Middletown, DE
17 August 2015